MODERATE DRINKING – NATURALLY!
Herbs and Vitamins to Control Your Drinking

Donna J. Cornett, M.A.

People Friendly Books
Santa Rosa, California USA

MODERATE DRINKING - NATURALLY!
Herbs and Vitamins to Control Your Drinking

People Friendly Books

For information address:
People Friendly Books
P.O. Box 5441
Santa Rosa, CA 95402
www.ModerateDrinkingPrograms.com
www.drinklinkmoderation.com

ISBN: 0-9763720-3-7

Printed in the United States of America

Library of Congress Control Number: 2006903671

To Darla, my sister with a heart of gold, who takes good care of everyone
To Dixie, my sister, whose courage awes me
To Dale, my sister, who inspires me

CONTENTS

Introduction

What is alcohol craving? What triggers it? How can you tame it? Do ancient medical systems offer treatments to prevent alcohol craving and alcohol abuse? Do Homeopathic, Chinese and Ayurvedic healers prescribe remedies to control drinking desire and alcohol consumption? What about European and Native American herbs, nutritional supplements and lifestyle adjustments? I've been asking myself these questions for years. After digging for the answers and finding only bits and pieces here and there, I decided to tackle these subjects so I wrote this book exploring complementary and alternative herbal remedies from around the world to reduce alcohol craving and consumption.

I think *Moderate Drinking - Naturally!* is a breakthrough for drinkers, alcohol abuse and health care professionals. It gives drinkers their first serious look into alternative medicine to control drinking desire and drinking. It fills a void in the traditional alcohol abuse prevention and treatment fields and lays the foundation for a natural school featuring organic options to prevent alcoholism. And it equips healthcare professionals with attractive new tools encouraging drinkers to seek early treatment for problem drinking. Hard to believe so little attention has been paid to alternative medicine to fight alcohol abuse!

What sparked my interest in alternative alcohol abuse treatment? I've always been fascinated with human behavior and been a big fan of complementary and alternative medicine. Then, after earning a couple of degrees in psychology, I felt I was drinking too much and I developed the Drink/Link Moderate Drinking Program in 1988. Drink/Link is a commonsense program teaching drinkers clinically-proven behavior management skills to improve drinking habits and attitudes, reduce alcohol consumption and prevent alcoholism.

After so many years of treating people with drinking problems, I began to focus on alcohol craving. I concluded "desire", "urge" or "craving" was the driving force behind that first drink and overdrinking and the bottom line to making a real difference in a person's drinking behavior was to address their alcohol craving. If you could control drinking desire, you could control drinking, avoid alcoholism and all of the health, relationship, workplace, legal and financial problems associated with it. And because of my interest in alternative medicine, it only seemed logical to look into natural options – not pharmaceuticals – to address it.

The more I thought about it, the more I was convinced offering natural remedies to reduce craving and consumption would be a great alcohol abuse prevention and treatment strategy too. So many people are attracted to alternative medicine – eighty percent of people worldwide use herbs for primary care purposes according to the World Health Organization – why not reach out to the millions of drinkers not interested in conventional alcohol abuse treatment and offer them herbal and nutritional tips to manage drinking? Enticing drinkers into early treatment with convenient, affordable, natural alternatives will dramatically lower the alcohol abuse rate.

When I first started writing this book I only investigated remedies to treat alcohol craving. But halfway through I decided I could not do justice to the subject unless I looked at the big picture and the physiological, psychological and spiritual factors which strongly influence craving. Common to many ancient medical systems, the concept of balance is the belief that equalizing the physical, mental and spiritual aspects of one's life is essential for and promotes good health. I think it is the antidote to alcohol craving and problem drinking too. If you feel good physically, mentally and spiritually, you don't need alcohol to feel better. That's why I also decided to offer remedies to nurture these three aspects of life – helping you to achieve harmonious living. Spreading the concept of balance to drinkers everywhere and encouraging physiological and psychological wellness so there is no need to drink is my mission these days.

This book has been an enlightening experience for me and I hope it's an enlightening experience for my colleagues in the traditional alcohol abuse research and treatment fields as well. For years researchers have been obsessed with isolating the "gene" for alcoholism and producing quick-fix "miracle" drugs to eliminate alcohol craving. Well, they are still looking for the alcoholism gene and many anti-alcohol drugs come with unwanted side effects or only work for a few people. How about some serious research into Mother Nature's pharmacy to help drinkers? Conventional alcohol abuse treatment needs a fresh, new approach too. It has prescribed abstinence and the 12 Step program for anyone with a drinking problem since the 1930's. And even though standard treatment has helped some, most drinkers never consider it because they don't feel their drinking is serious enough to quit, support group meetings don't appeal to them or they can't buy the concept of a "higher power." Researching and offering drinkers natural options to prevent alcohol abuse is long overdue.

Finally, I hope *Moderate Drinking - Naturally!* is an enlightening experience for you too. Motivating you to take control of your drinking sooner rather than later, so you don't graduate to alcoholism. Encouraging you to examine the cues that trigger your alcohol craving and arming yourself with skills and strategies that will help you to stay within moderate drinking limits. And always striving for a balanced lifestyle so moderation in all things comes easily to you.

Welcome to the brave new world of alternative alcohol abuse treatment! I hope you find these tips as fascinating as I do.

Cheers,

Donna Cornett
Founder & Director
Drink/Link Moderate Drinking Programs & Products
www.ModerateDrinkingPrograms.com
www.drinklinkmoderation.com
Telephone: 707-539-5465
Toll-free: 888-773-7465
Fax: 707-537-1010
P.O. Box 5441
Santa Rosa, California 95402 USA

P. S. Moderate Drinking - Naturally! Volume Two is in the works – exploring even more alternative methods to outsmart craving and achieve balance. Look for it.

DISCLAIMER

The information in this book has not been evaluated by the United States Food and Drug Administration. The information contained in this book is for educational and entertainment purposes only and is not intended for diagnosing, treating, curing or preventing any illness. The author does not directly or indirectly offer medical advice, prescribe nutritional or herbal remedies or assume any responsibility for anyone who chooses to treat themselves with the medicines listed here. The author cannot accept responsibility for any consequences, injury or damage to a person or property from the misuse of information contained in this book.

The United States Food and Drug Administration does not fully regulate the manufacturing and sale of herbal and nutritional dietary supplements. Many herbal and nutritional supplements, especially when not used correctly, could pose a serious health risk. Some could exacerbate a pre-existing medical or psychological condition and interact with over-the-counter and prescription medications resulting in death. The reader is advised to consult their healthcare provider, physician, licensed or qualified alternative medicine practitioner, nurse or pharmacist for correct prescription, dosage, precautions, side effects and interactions before experimenting with any dietary supplement.

This book is not recommended for the alcoholic, anyone experiencing serious health, psychological, social, workplace, legal or financial problems as a result of alcohol use or anyone suffering from a physical and/or psychological condition aggravated by alcohol consumption. It is not recommended for any woman who is pregnant or may become pregnant, any minor or anyone who has successfully abstained from alcohol. Results vary according to the individual.

Finally, note that alcohol withdrawal and detoxification can be life threatening and require medical supervision. Remedies in this book do not replace the medical supervision needed to treat an individual undergoing alcohol withdrawal and detoxification.

MODERATE DRINKING - NATURALLY!

Part One:
FOR YOUR INFORMATION . . .

Chapter 1
Words to the Wise

Alcoholic beverages have been around for at least 12,000 years. "Bread and beer," was a common greeting for the ancient Egyptians. About 1100 BC, the Chinese proclaimed moderate alcohol use was required by heaven. "He was a wise man who invented beer," declared Plato. Jesus drank and approved of drinking in moderation. Early Christians thought alcohol was a gift from God and to scorn it was heresy. And Ben Franklin believed, "Beer is proof God loves us and wants us to be happy." People everywhere have been singing the praises of moderate drinking for centuries.

Unfortunately, alcohol abuse is as old as alcohol use. And craving alcohol too much and too often can get you in trouble. In fact, research shows alcohol craving is linked to alcohol consumption – the more you crave, the more you drink and the greater your chances of developing a drinking problem.

If you think you're becoming a slave to drinking desire, this book may be for you. With it you'll learn about all-natural commonsense tips and nutritional and herbal remedies to reduce alcohol craving and consumption. And you'll also explore vitamin and botanical aids to help you pave the way to physical, mental and spiritual balance – leading to overall good health and less need for alcohol.

We'll start by examining lifestyle issues and drinking triggers. Next, we'll look into nutritional supplements, traditional European and Native American herbs and Homeopathic medicine. Then we'll unearth Chinese and Ayurvedic remedies. Most chapters are divided into three sections. First, we look into preparations to detoxify and relieve withdrawal symptoms. Cleaning and healing the liver, blood and body promotes physical health and increases energy. The second section of the chapter investigates ways to calm the nerves and brighten the mood – encouraging psychological and spiritual wellness. And the third section of the chapter covers remedies targeting alcohol craving specifically.

But a little knowledge is a dangerous thing, so before you embark on this great adventure you must understand who this book is for, key terms which will be used throughout the book, exactly what this book does and does not cover and pointers on how to derive the greatest benefits from complementary and alternative medicine.

Who Are We Talking To?

You! If you are one of the millions of health-conscious drinkers eager to reduce your alcohol craving and consumption. It is also for alcohol abuse professionals and alternative and western medicine practitioners interested in natural treatments. And let's not forget anyone concerned about healthcare and alternative medicine in general.

The information contained in this book is not recommended for the alcoholic or anyone experiencing serious health, psychological, social, workplace, legal or financial problems because of alcohol use. If you suffer from a mental or medical problem or take any medication, treatments in this book could pose a serious health risk to you. They may exacerbate a pre-existing health or psychological condition and interact with other drugs which may be life threatening. This book is not intended to diagnose, treat, cure or prevent any illness and does not replace medical supervision required for alcohol withdrawal and detoxification.

What Are We Talking About?

We will talk about "natural remedies" and "alternative" and "complementary" medicine throughout this book. Here we will define "natural remedy" as a dietary supplement made of substances produced or existing in nature. The U.S. Food and Drug Administration defines a dietary supplement as a product taken orally that contains a "dietary ingredient" and is meant to supplement the diet. Dietary ingredients include vitamins, minerals, amino acids, herbs or other botanicals, enzymes, organ tissues, glandulars and metabolites.

Now let's turn our attention to the National Center for Complementary and Alternative Medicine (NCCAM), which is the United States government lead agency for scientific research on complementary and alternative medicine (CAM). According to NCCAM, "alternative" and "complementary" medicine is a "group of diverse medical and health care systems, practices and products that are not presently considered to be part of conventional medicine." "Complementary medicine" is used together with conventional medicine. And "alternative medicine" is used in place of conventional medicine. Complementary and alternative remedies which are not considered a part of conventional western medicine are covered here.

FYI – NCCAM's mission is to support research on complementary and alternative healing practices, train CAM researchers and to inform the public and health professionals about CAM therapies that work, do not work and why. One of their goals is to evaluate the safety and effectiveness of herbs and nutritional substances – many contained in this book. For more information about NCCAM, log on to their website at http://nccam.nih.gov.

So many natural remedies, so little time. Since there are hundreds of CAM systems worldwide, we must limit ourselves to the most popular ones. With a few exceptions, we must also limit ourselves to single herbs, plants, minerals, animal products and nutritional supplements. There is no time or space for the thousands of combinations or formulas on the market.

It seems every alternative medicine practitioner has a different take on which nutritional and herbal supplements work best to detoxify, improve mood and reduce alcohol craving. We have done our best to stay true to the spirit of each medical system by listing the most widely used remedies within that system to achieve these goals. Also keep in mind many of the medicines offered here do not have scientific proof to support claims made about them and the uses of many preparations are based on observation and anecdotal evidence provided by alternative medicine practitioners.

The remedies in this book are listed in alphabetical order, not in the order of their importance. You may see the same herb listed in two or more medical systems. And the same herb may be used in different systems to treat the same symptoms or different symptoms. It may also be given to treat several symptoms. For example, dandelion is prescribed in both European and Chinese herbal medicine to detoxify the body and St. John's wort is considered an excellent antidepressant in addition to being an anti-craving agent.

Most of the preparations listed here are derived from plants and have at least two names – the common English name and the botanical name. Ayurvedic herbs are known by four different names! Botanical, English, Sanskrit and Hindi. It can get pretty confusing. Here the common English name and the botanical name for each herb is given.

Remember – this book is intended to be educational and entertaining. It is not a self-help book because it does not provide specific dosage or preparation instructions. Prescription, dosage and preparation for each medicine varies according to the individual. Some of these remedies can make you very sick or even be fatal if they are not properly prescribed or if you take the wrong dosage. Professional guidance is a must if you are interested in experimenting with any of these substances. Assume full responsibility for your actions if you try any remedy on your own without professional supervision.

No Magic Bullets Here!

Even though lifestyle, herbal and nutritional tips in this book may lessen your need for alcohol – making it easier for you to learn safe-drinking habits – they are not "magic bullets" which will automatically correct unhealthy attitudes and behaviors you have formed around drinking and alcohol over the years. To get the most from these tips, which are only a small but helpful part of the safe-drinking equation, you must also learn and practice sensible drinking skills.

Marlatt and Gordon, two highly-respected researchers in the alcohol abuse prevention and treatment fields, believe a drinker must be proactive to improve drinking behavior. Marlatt offers several commonsense suggestions to do just that. First, you must modify your lifestyle to better deal with stress and high-risk drinking situations. Second, you must identify and respond appropriately to cues that trigger destructive drinking patterns. And third, you must practice behavior management strategies to reduce the risk of reverting back to problem drinking habits. Amen!

To learn more about moderate drinking strategies and techniques, contact Drink/Link Moderate Drinking Programs & Products at www.ModerateDrinkingPrograms.com or call 888-773-7465 to purchase the Self-Study or Telephone Counseling Program. Or pick up the book *7 Weeks to Safe Social Drinking: How to Effectively Moderate Your Alcohol*

Intake by Donna J. Cornett. The programs and book teach you clinically-proven behavior management skills to pace your drinking, reduce alcohol consumption and prevent alcoholism.

How Can You Get the Most From CAM Remedies?

Start by evaluating the state of your health and any pre-existing medical or psychological condition you may suffer from before considering any CAM treatments. Doctors are taught "first do no harm" when treating a patient. Apply that philosophy to yourself.

Second, if you are interested in trying any CAM therapy discuss it with your trusted physician first. He or she will be able to warn you if the remedy you are interested in is not right for you – aggravating a health or psychological condition or interacting with medications you may be taking.

Third, consult a licensed or qualified CAM practitioner in the area of your interest for correct prescription and dosage. Some herbs may be toxic – even fatal – if not properly prescribed. You want to reap the benefits of alternative medicine, not kill yourself! And when looking for a licensed or qualified practitioner examine their credentials and beware of any unrealistic claims they make. Problem-free drinking in seven days? Impossible. If what they offer sounds too good to be true, it probably is.

Fourth, if you assume the responsibility of experimenting with any medicine become an informed consumer. Investigate the safety of the remedy, the scientific evidence backing its effectiveness and check for precautions, warnings, side effects and interactions.

Fifth, get the purest and most refined form of the product you are thinking about. Where and how was the supplement processed? Read the label to see if any other ingredients were added. The more refined the remedy, the more likely it will achieve the desired effect and the less likely it will produce unwanted side effects. A qualified CAM practitioner specializing in the therapy you are interested in can direct you to the purest products on the market.

Sixth, if you do experiment with CAM medicines try only one at a time. Herbal interactions may be hazardous to your health and interfere with a preparation's effectiveness. Besides, you won't know which one is working for you.

Seventh, if you experience any unpleasant side effects discontinue use of the remedy immediately. Each one of us has been blessed with a unique metabolism. That means different people react to different things in different ways. If you have any negative reactions to any substance, just stop!

And Enjoy the Ride. . .

For fun, the Craving Game – a little exercise designed to help you learn more about your desire to drink, your drinking habits and yourself – will conclude every chapter. Complete it. It's just another tool to heighten your "alcohol craving awareness" – and to make it easier for you to stay on the moderate drinking track.

Chapter 2

Could You Transform Your Life
If You Tamed Your Desire to Drink?

Think of it . . . No longer being a slave to alcohol craving. No longer wrestling with a strong desire to start drinking. No longer continuing to drink until you're drunk. No longer assigning such great importance to alcohol and drinking.

Drinking sensibly each and every time and never worrying about going overboard. Putting alcohol in perspective, so your life does not revolve around that first drink of the day. A drink or two is not a necessity but a complement to your healthy lifestyle. And enjoying the peace of mind that comes with guilt-free, problem-free drinking. How could you transform your life if you tamed your desire to drink and stuck to moderate drinking habits?

But before you get going on the changes you need to make, you must first determine if you have a drinking problem and how serious it is. Then weigh the positives of moderate drinking versus the negatives of problem drinking to get yourself motivated for the transformation ahead.

What is a "Drinking Problem"?

Alcohol abuse and alcoholism are both considered "drinking problems." There are many definitions for each term – some include alcohol craving as a symptom and some do not. Generally speaking, if you are troubled by any health, relationship, social, work, legal or financial problems because of drinking, you have a "drinking problem."

Now let's get specific. According to the American Psychiatric Association, a person suffering from alcohol abuse or "problem drinking" displays one or more of the following symptoms within a 12-month period:

- Failure to meet work, school or home obligations because of recurrent alcohol use
- Placing yourself in physically dangerous situations, like drinking and driving, because of recurrent alcohol use
- Legal problems resulting from recurrent alcohol use
- Continuing to drink alcohol despite social or interpersonal problems resulting from alcohol use

If you are experiencing one or more of these symptoms, the bad news is you are a problem drinker. But the good news is you are still capable of modifying your drinking habits and returning to problem-free moderate drinking with the right tools.

What is a serious drinking problem? According to the American Psychiatric Association, a person suffering from alcohol dependence or "alcoholism" displays three or more of the following symptoms within a 12-month period:

- The need to drink more and more alcohol to get high
- Drinking more alcohol or over a longer period of time than you intend
- Experiencing physical withdrawal symptoms, like stomach upset, headache, sweating, rapid pulse rate, tremors, insomnia or anxiety, if you reduce or stop alcohol intake

- A desire or failed attempts to reduce or control your drinking
- Spending too much time obtaining alcohol, drinking alcohol and recovering from alcohol
- Limiting recreational, social or occupational activities because of alcohol
- Continued drinking despite ongoing physical or psychological problems caused or aggravated by alcohol use

If you are living with three or more of these symptoms, you are an alcoholic and trying to control craving and drinking would be difficult, if not impossible. You have a serious drinking problem and need to stop. One or two remedies from this book will not help you to manage alcohol.

Consider These Cold, Hard Facts
Over Your Next Drink . . .

Next to smoking, alcohol abuse is the second leading cause of preventable death in the United States. Over one hundred thousand deaths a year can be blamed on alcohol, according to the National Council on Alcohol and Drug Dependence. If you are an alcoholic, take ten to twelve years off of your life expectancy. And that's just for starters.

Chronic, heavy drinking harms all the tissues and organs in your body. It weakens the immune system and dramatically increases your chances of developing liver, heart, gastrointestinal and upper digestive tract diseases.

Alcohol abuse is the leading cause of illness and death from liver disease – more than two million people in the United States suffer from alcohol-related liver disease. Your risk of developing alcoholic hepatitis (inflammation of the liver), cirrhosis of the liver (scarring of the liver) and liver cancer, especially if you suffer from the hepatitis C virus, significantly increase the more you drink. Each one of these liver diseases may result in death if not treated.

Heart problems caused by heavy alcohol consumption include cardiomyopathy and arrhythmias. Hypertension and stroke are also associated with too much booze. The odds of developing stomach and intestinal diseases, including pancreatitis, dramatically increase the more you drink. And your chances of developing cancer of the mouth, throat, esophagus, larynx, colon and rectum also rise with increased alcohol consumption. If you drink when you are pregnant, you put your baby at risk for birth defects, including fetal alcohol syndrome – a condition characterized by severe physical, mental and behavioral problems.

Health costs for alcoholics are much higher than for non-alcoholics. Twenty-five to forty percent of all patients admitted to hospitals in this country are treated for alcohol-related problems! According to the National Institute on Alcohol Abuse and Alcoholism, half of all fatal car accidents, forty-one percent of all crimes, fifty percent of all homicides, one third of all suicides and a large number of drowning, aviation and boating deaths can be blamed on alcohol. Alcohol abuse is also linked to domestic violence and often plays a role in workplace injuries and fatalities.

These cold, hard facts should make you think twice about overdrinking . . .

How Has Alcohol Affected Your Life?

Now let's get personal. How many alcohol-related problems are you dealing with? Too many hangovers, headaches or stomachaches after partying? Suffering from health problems, like high blood pressure, pancreas or liver disease? Has your doctor ever advised you to cut down or quit drinking?

How about family problems? Does your significant other nag you about how much you drink? Are you constantly fighting over your alcohol use? Is your mate threatening separation or divorce if you don't get a grip on your drinking? Do you become verbally abusive when you drink too much? Or a TV-watching, couch potato always with a drink in your hand?

Not meeting important family obligations because of liquor? Like picking up the kids from school on time or making their soccer games. Would you rather be drinking instead? Are your children embarrassed by you when you drink? Have they stopped inviting their friends to the house because of your alcohol habit? Do you feel you are a failure as a parent and role model because of booze? Drinking may be getting in the way of one the most important areas of your life – a happy family.

Do friends comment on how aggressive and belligerent you get after one too many? Do you become brutally honest or blow up when under the influence? Then rush to apologize the next day because you were out of line? Or do you black out and don't even remember your off-the-wall drinking behavior?

Problems at work because of alcohol? Are you in hot water over poor job performance? Is your career on the line because you've been late or called in sick too many times? Ever been fired because you were a no-show once too often? Serious work and financial problems caused by alcohol are real wake-up calls.

Any legal consequences because of drinking? Any DUI's or DWI's requiring high-priced lawyers to get you off the hook? Ever been arrested for public drunkenness or disturbing the peace? Costly symptoms of alcohol abuse which can drain the pocketbook.

Do you feel guilty and ashamed of your out-of-control drinking behavior? Has your self-esteem and self-confidence evaporated in alcohol? Is your good reputation, which is so precious to you, being soiled with each destructive drinking episode? Are you earning the reputation of being a pathetic lush who can't hold your liquor?

If you are suffering from any of these problems, you are an alcohol abuser. And it's time you sat up, took notice and committed to a moderate drinking plan. Catch yourself before you fall . . .

How Good Could Your Life Get with Less Alcohol?

You'd feel a lot better in the morning to start with. Perky and well-rested – no hangover or headache. Not slow from too much booze the night before. And tons more energy in general – for family, for work, for living!

Drinking less clears the alcohol-related fog from your brain. You feel healthy, physically and mentally, and you're enjoying a positive outlook. And you feel confident and in control – now that alcohol is no longer holding you back.

Your mate and family notice a difference in you too. They like you so much better when you stay within reasonable drinking limits. Fewer arguments and no more nagging about booze. It's no longer an issue between you and your mate. Alcohol is no longer an obstacle to a healthy relationship.

And family matters again – now that you aren't distracted by alcohol. Instead of being the old couch potato focused on drinking and TV, now you are investing time and energy in the kids and family. Your children see the fine role model you have always wanted to be – a responsible adult, caring parent and sensible drinker. They are no longer ashamed and embarrassed by you and feel comfortable inviting their friends to the house now that your drinking is under control. You will regain your kids respect when you manage alcohol like an adult.

Your friends appreciate the positive changes they see in you too. No more flying off the handle at the smallest thing – like when you were drinking heavily. No more standing them up in favor of alcohol. They no longer have to keep an eye on you – making sure you get home safely after a party. You are no longer a burden to your friends. People you like, like your moderate drinking ways.

The job and colleagues are working out too. The boss notices you're turning over a new leaf – attendance is excellent and productivity is soaring. You have the energy to devote to a good day's work and you take pride in it. You feel ambitious and look forward to the next level and more money because alcohol is no longer sapping your energy.

You will start to like yourself again and take back your precious reputation too. Liquor is no longer interfering with the fine person you really are. You are rebuilding your self-esteem and reputation – from loser to respected adult when you keep alcohol in check. And your mate, your family, your friends and your colleagues look up to you – when you're on the safe-drinking track. Great reasons to get excited about moderate drinking.

Better yet, you will enjoy the peace of mind that comes from no longer worrying about your problem drinking. No more fears about your health or losing your family because of booze. No more shame about your behavior. You are no longer concerned you'll lose your job or drive drunk. Or about legal tangles and costly lawyers because of alcohol.

A great burden will be lifted off of your shoulders when problem drinking no longer factors into your life. Commit yourself to moderate drinking and live the life you've always dreamed of . . .

The Craving Game

Could you transform your life if you curbed alcohol craving and drank less? Sit down and make two lists. One list of the negative consequences of your drinking and another list of the positive consequences of moderate drinking.

Now on a scale from one to ten, with one being least motivated and ten being highly motivated, how eager are you to tackle drinking desire? If you are highly motivated – six or higher – chances are good you'll drink less.

Getting pumped up is the first step to changing drinking attitudes and behaviors. From now on, reflect on all of the positives of moderate drinking and how you will transform your life when you drink sensibly.

Chapter 3
What is Alcohol Craving?

To drink or not to drink? Kevin was fighting a red hot craving for his first cocktail of the day. His overwhelming desire for a martini after work versus his recent commitment to kick a growing drinking habit was a real dilemma. He realized that powerful urge to drink at the same time, the same place and for the same reasons would make cutting back tough.

Kevin's daily routine was filled with obstacles challenging his moderate drinking goal. After work, around seven in the evening, was the first hurdle. A little bell rang in his head when he left the office telling him cocktail hour was right around the corner. Literally, right around the corner from his office was the lounge he dropped by most nights after work to unwind with a drink. He was friendly with the barflies and the bartender, who not only served up a great martini but a good joke too.

Ahhh . . . the sight and smell of that first martini – two olives please – before it even touched his lips. That first sip made his day. He knew he could kiss off his troubles because the alcohol would soon be kicking in. Two or three or four martinis later and it was a party.

Those were the good old days. But the last couple of months he felt his need to drink and his drinking were getting out of hand. Sometimes he would skip dinner in favor of drinking and nurse a hangover the next morning. Feeling slow affected his job performance the next day. He worried about the long-term health consequences of heavy drinking. Plus, his wife did not appreciate him spending more time with his martini at the bar than with her. His reputation at home and at work was on the line because of too much alcohol, not to mention the toll it was taking on his self-esteem and self-confidence.

What if Kevin no longer had to wrestle with an intense craving for alcohol? What if he could reduce or eliminate his drinking desire? Sticking to a moderate drinking plan would certainly be easier. He would no longer be chained to an alcohol habit or agonize over the "drink or not to drink" dilemma. Or worry about out-of-control drinking, hangovers, health problems, being labeled a lush or graduating to alcoholism. And let's not overlook improved relations with his wife and taking pride in himself again.

Many experts believe alcohol craving leads to the development and maintenance of problem drinking. And if you could reduce drinking desire, you could reduce alcohol consumption. Time to take a closer look at what craving is, how it works and what triggers it before you tackle it with natural remedies.

Definitions and Aspects of Alcohol Craving

Alcohol craving was first recognized as a symptom of alcoholism by E. M. Jellinek and colleagues in 1955. It's amazing it took so long to get noticed since many felt it played a major role in the development of alcoholism. Researchers lost interest in the subject for years. Then in the 1990's, alcohol craving became a hot topic again.

Desire, urge, need, longing, yearning, hankering, appetite, hunger, passion, want. The National Institute on Alcohol Abuse and Alcoholism defines alcohol craving as "a strong need, or compulsion, to drink." Others describe it as "intense thoughts about alcohol." To date, there is still no one common definition of alcohol craving agreed upon by clinicians and researchers. But most do agree it is an important factor associated with loss of control, alcoholism and relapsing back to destructive drinking behavior.

Why do people crave alcohol? Some drink to ease stress and to relax. Some drink to relieve physiological or psychological pain. And some people drink to fight off withdrawal symptoms brought on by reducing or stopping drinking. Mild craving is characterized by psychological and/or physiological tension, uneasiness or irritability. Strong craving is characterized by more powerful feelings – psychological and/or physiological apprehension or distress.

A highly complex phenomenon, alcohol craving may be conscious or unconscious. It may occur spontaneously or be triggered by internal or external cues. It could be psychological or physiological or both. Psychological craving is a nagging desire to give in and start drinking. Problem drinkers often suffer from a psychological craving to drink. If alcohol is needed to fend off withdrawal symptoms – like a headache, stomachache, shaky hands, irritability or insomnia because one has cut down or stopped drinking – it is a sign of physiological craving. Alcoholics suffer from both psychological and physiological cravings.

A subjective feeling for each individual, some experts believe alcohol craving is an emotion. Others see it as a cycle. Like a wave on the beach – starting small, gaining in strength, peaking, and then fading. A wave of thoughts and feelings about alcohol and drinking that become stronger and stronger then melt away.

Even though there is a lot of speculation about what alcohol craving is and how it comes about, one thing is certain: the greater the urge to drink, the more difficult it is to resist alcohol – which could lead to problem drinking.

Alcohol, Your Brain and Craving

Alcohol craving occurs as a result of a complicated set of interactions between certain brain structures and brain chemistry. The "reward center" or nucleus accumbens, the amygdala which regulates mood and stress, the basal ganglia which affects behavior and thought patterns and the dorsal lateral prefrontal cortex which stores positive memories of alcohol use all work together in the brain to produce drinking desire.

It is believed alcohol activates the reward center and reinforces drinking by sending information to these other brain structures involved with memory, emotions and learning – all factors involved in alcohol craving.

Measuring Your Craving

Measuring alcohol craving is not an exact science. Many studies looking into craving simply ask the drinker to rate the intensity of their craving. Some involve scales with questions or statements covering different aspects of craving. Others observe physiological variations in heart rate, blood pressure or sweat gland activity, even though it has been concluded these physiological changes may not necessarily be associated with craving. Observing a person's behavior, including how long they drink, how many drinks they consume and the time between exposure to cues and the onset of drinking, is yet another means of assessing craving.

So Many Alcohol Craving Theories, So Little Time . . .

There are many theoretical models explaining alcohol craving, but most can be classified as either conditioning or cognitive models. Conditioning theories argue if you repeatedly pair alcohol-related cues (like the sight or smell of your favorite drink) with drinking alcohol, these cues then become "conditioned stimuli" and produce the same physiological and psychological responses you experience when you actually drink alcohol. Craving occurs if you do not drink immediately when experiencing conditioned stimuli responses.

Cognitive theories of alcohol craving assume thought processes are involved in your reactions to alcohol and alcohol-related cues. Over the years you have formed positive memories, beliefs and expectations about alcohol and drinking. Craving occurs because of these memories, beliefs and expectations – especially if you make a conscious effort to avoid drinking.

Then there is the neuroadaptive model of alcohol craving which states changes in the nervous system caused by years of alcohol abuse lead to craving. The body adapts to the constant presence of alcohol and it is needed to feel normal and to maintain vital physiological functions, like blood pressure and body temperature. Without alcohol, the drinker suffers physiological and psychological stress. Craving occurs to maintain the normal state of the body and to ward off withdrawal symptoms.

Many believe neurotransmitters – powerful chemicals in the brain that are natural painkillers and mood enhancers – are responsible for alcohol craving. They think neurotransmitter deficiencies may initiate craving. If these deficiencies are restored however, brain chemistry returns to normal and craving wanes.

Still others believe low blood sugar levels or hypoglycemia account for alcohol craving. They think craving occurs to normalize blood sugar levels in the body.

What aspects of these alcohol craving theories may apply to your drinking desire?

What Cues Trigger Your Desire to Drink?

If you recognize the cues triggering your alcohol craving, you will defuse the power of the craving, be less susceptible to it and be less likely to slip into problem drinking habits. Craving awareness is a beautiful thing!

External cues which may trigger drinking desire might include people, places, things, environments. Keeping company with a heavy-drinking crowd who always has liquor on hand and encourages you to drink. Your favorite drinking place – a club, restaurant or your home. The mere sight or smell of beer, wine or spirits may spark your need to drink. Or social occasions might be your downfall.

Internal cues involving physiological needs and states of mind can also be powerful triggers. Thirst, hunger, fatigue and pain may start you craving. Emotions can trip drinking desire too. Celebrating with a drinking party or drowning your sorrows in booze. Anger, frustration, depression, stress, mood and anxiety disorders, including panic attacks, post-traumatic stress syndrome, obsessive-compulsive behavior, bipolar and social disorders, can all lead to alcohol craving and abuse. Positive memories, beliefs and expectations surrounding alcohol also come into the mix when examining craving cues.

If you think you suffer from a health or psychiatric disorder, it is crucial you seek professional help to address the problem so you can feel better without alcohol.

The Craving Game

Start a Craving Diary to heighten your craving awareness. Every time the urge to drink strikes, whether it's your first drink of the day, second or third, rate your craving on a scale from one to ten. Number one being the least intense craving and number ten being the most intense craving. Where do you fall? Record the intensity of every craving from now on.

Keeping track of your drinking desire will not only sharpen your craving awareness, it will also help you gain insight into the important role it plays in your drinking behavior.

Part Two:
COMMONSENSE TOOLS
TO BEAT ALCOHOL CRAVING

Chapter 4

A Healthy Lifestyle is the Antidote to Alcohol Appetite

If you feel great physically, mentally and spiritually, the less you will need alcohol. This chapter gives you tips to do just that – focusing on healthy living habits and attitudes. Your body is a temple. Worship it and let go of the desire to drink . . .

"Let thy food be thy medicine and thy medicine be thy food" – Hippocrates

A nutritious diet with lots of fruits, vegetables, grains and dairy, light on meat with just a touch of fat is the medicine that will stabilize your blood sugar, increase your energy, promote feelings of well-being and decrease your alcohol appetite.

The 2005 Dietary Guidelines for Americans, developed jointly by the U.S. Departments of Agriculture and Health and Human Services, outlines exactly what a healthy diet is. In a nutshell, they recommend you eat plenty of fruits, vegetables and whole grains plus milk or milk products each day. Two cups of fruit – mangoes, bananas, oranges, grapes, apples, pineapple, papaya, strawberries, peaches or kiwi fruit. Two and one-half cups of vegetables – broccoli, carrots, squash, dried beans, tofu, potatoes, corn, peas, tomatoes, lettuce or green beans. Three or more ounces of whole-grain products, like wild rice, popcorn, whole wheat bread, brown rice or oatmeal, and three cups of fat-free or low-fat milk or milk products will round out your healthy diet every day.

Try to make plant foods – fruits, vegetables and grains – the foundation of your diet. You'll get most of the nutrients you need from a plant-based diet and avoid saturated fat, cholesterol and sodium. Add your dairy products, a little meat and olive oil on the side and voila! You are well on your way to better eating and better health.

Also take to heart nutritional advice specifically for people cutting back on alcohol. Eating less sugar and high-fat fried foods, including junk food, drinking less caffeine and increasing complex carbohydrates like grains, beans and veggies may be your meal ticket to beating the alcohol habit, according to some experts. Research shows sugar, caffeine and fatty fried foods are linked to alcohol craving and increase the desire to drink. One 1991 study, which restricted sugar, eliminated caffeine and increased complex carbohydrates, showed decreased alcohol craving in drinkers. In a 1983 study, some drinkers were given a hospital diet and some were given a special diet, which included fruits and wheat germ, but excluded coffee, dairy products, junk food and peanut butter. Six months later, less than thirty-eight percent of the drinkers on the hospital diet remained abstinent compared to eighty-one percent of the drinkers on the special diet. Animal studies have also shown diets loaded with junk food increase alcohol consumption.

On the other hand, some professionals emphasize the importance of eating three protein-packed meals a day to restore a protein deficiency individuals with substance abuse problems often suffer from. They believe extra protein stabilizes blood sugar and mood, making reducing or stopping drinking easier.

Eat healthy and notice a difference in your physical and mental outlook within days. For more information on the Dietary Guidelines for Americans, logon to www.healthierus.gov/dietary guidelines.

"Movement is a medicine for creating change in a person's physical, emotional and mental states" – Carol Welch

To create a change in your drinking desire, exercise must be on your agenda. It builds and maintains healthy bones, muscles and joints. It helps you to lose or manage weight and increases endurance and muscle strength. Exercise lowers your risk for high blood pressure, cardiovascular disease, colon cancer and diabetes, to name just a few of the health benefits. Psychologically, it has been proven to reduce stress, anxiety and depression and increase feelings of well-being and self-esteem. Exercise not only takes the edge off of your alcohol appetite, it limits your drinking time too. It's impossible to drink while you're doing crunches!

Just thirty minutes of physical activity a day, most days of the week, and you will notice positive physiological and psychological changes within a week or two. First, look at ways you can easily incorporate exercise into your daily routine. Get out of the car and walk or bicycle to your destination. Forget the elevator and walk up stairs. Get rid of the polluting power mower and use a push mower instead. Play with the kids or clean the house. Garden. Exercise or pedal your stationary bike while listening to music or watching TV. Walk the dog. Brainstorm all the ways you can pump up your activity level naturally by making simple adjustments to your routine. They all count as part of your thirty-minute exercise commitment.

Or go out of your way with planned exercise. Brisk walking, bicycling or jogging. Add thirty minutes of swimming, golfing, ice skating or basketball each day and watch the pounds melt away. Take a yoga, aerobics or dance class. Who knows? You might even achieve a "runner's high" – a release of endorphins in your bloodstream which produces a great mood and lust for life.

Check with your physician before you start pumping up – especially if you have any pre-existing health problems.

"Sleep is the golden chain that ties health and our bodies together" – Thomas Dekker

Study after study shows most of us suffer from sleep deprivation – making us feel tired, irritable and unable to concentrate on the day's activities. It may also increase your need to drink – looking to alcohol to give you a quick pick-me-up. Commuting, working, taxiing kids, dinner, household chores and getting ready for the next day barely gives you a chance to think, let alone sleep. Five or six days a week of this schedule without much rest and you're ready to collapse at week's end.

Your goal should be seven or eight hours of restful sleep each night. If you're not getting that now, you need to make some changes – like planning on going to bed earlier or saving some chores for the weekend so you can fit in a solid eight hours.

Look at your schedule. Where can changes be made? Obviously, prioritize and get to the most important tasks of your day first. The rest can wait so you can get to bed earlier and wake up the next morning feeling relaxed, refreshed and focused.

Wrap yourself in the golden chain of sleep each night and watch the need to drink fade away.

"A good laugh and a long sleep are the best cures in the doctor's book" – Irish proverb

Playing and having fun is just as important as getting your rest, when it comes to reducing alcohol craving. Feeling stressed, isolated and concentrating only on your career, money and getting ahead makes you a dull person and more likely to turn to alcohol for a "fun fix." Get out, kick up your heels and have a good time. It may be just what the doctor orders to curb your drinking desire.

When was the last time you did something special – without alcohol? Solitary activities, like hiking, painting or museum hopping, will work. Or social events, like dinner with friends, dancing or a golf or tennis game, will do too. Liven up your life, reduce your stress level and watch your desire to drink diminish.

Remember – socializing does not necessarily require alcohol. If drinking is in the picture when you do party, focus on the people, the conversation and entertainment – not on the booze.

Commit to a good time at least twice a week and say goodbye to alcohol craving.

"Love yourself first and everything else falls into place" – Lucille Ball

The better you feel about yourself and the direction of your life, the less interested you will be in alcohol to improve your mood. On the flip side, the less you like yourself and the lower your self-esteem, the more inclined you will be to medicate with alcohol.

Self-esteem is the opinion you have of yourself. How do you feel about yourself? On a scale from one to ten, with one being the lowest self-esteem and ten being the strongest self-esteem, where do you fall?

Five or less and you are suffering from low self-esteem. Now comes the hard part. You must determine what is eating away at your self-image and fix it. Troubled relationships? Not getting ahead? Never graduated from college or promoted to your dream job? Not feeling appreciated by family, friends or colleagues?

Whatever the problem is, you need to recognize it, define it, consider different solutions to fix it and follow through with the best plan. This may mean changes in relationships. It may mean going back to school or pursuing the career you have always wanted. It may mean making more money or volunteering in your community. Or it may mean seeking the professional help of a psychologist, educational or career counselor to help you examine and overcome obstacles holding you back.

Love yourself first and watch moderate drinking fall into place.

"Look at the big picture and put alcohol in perspective – and you'll never worry about problem drinking again" – Donna Cornett

So many drinkers – especially problem drinkers – assign such great importance to alcohol and the role it plays in their lives. If you are one of those drinkers who feels passionately about alcohol, it's time for an attitude adjustment.

Pinch yourself every time you start thinking of alcohol or drinking. Remind yourself alcohol is not the be-all and end-all and spending too much time and energy obsessing about it is unhealthy and leads to problem drinking. Then reflect on the big picture of your life – family, friends, work and play. Alcohol and drinking are really insignificant in the scheme of things compared to the people and things that mean the most to you. And to risk any aspect of your wonderful life because of your love of alcohol would be silly.

Yes, a couple of drinks can enhance the quality of your life, but handing your power over to alcohol and abusing it could destroy you and the big picture. Put alcohol in perspective and watch craving wane.

The Craving Game

What lifestyle habits and attitudes do you need to brush up on? Better diet? More exercise? More rest? More fun? Increased self-esteem? An attitude adjustment about alcohol?

Write down specific plans to improve the quality of your life. For example, to improve your eating habits start your grocery shopping in the produce department and stock up there first. Or make a point of getting to bed one hour earlier weekday nights. Treat yourself to shopping spree or make a dinner date for a good time. And every time you think of alcohol, think about how unimportant it really is in the big picture. Your payoff is reduced alcohol craving!

Chapter 5
Amazing Commonsense Tips to Curb Drinking Desire

What triggers your desire to drink? What if you could manage these drinking cues so they would no longer lead to alcohol craving and problem drinking? This chapter looks into environmental, physiological and psychological drinking cues and how you can handle them so you don't fall into the old drinking trap. Bonus anti-craving, moderate drinking suggestions round out the chapter.

Environmental Cues

The Sight and Smell of Alcohol

That's the bait. Just the sight of your favorite drink gets you going. Start craving alcohol that is. You have been well-conditioned to your drink of choice just as Pavlov's dog was to a bell.

Cassie was conditioned to the sight of fine wines. She lives in the California wine country and is surrounded by vineyards, wineries and restaurants offering premium wines. She had a huge wine rack in her kitchen stacked with the best. Passing by the rack, especially in the late afternoon, she sometimes felt tempted to alter her plans for the day and pour herself a glass of red wine instead. Occasionally, she gave into this desire. But she was not happy with herself when she started drinking too early in the day, so she decided to eliminate this cue and put the wine rack in the garage. Out of sight, out of mind. No more visual cue and a lot less temptation meant less drinking for Cassie.

Another challenge for Cassie was being around an opened bottle of wine and watching other drinkers swirling, sniffing, sipping and enjoying their glasses. That whetted her appetite for a taste too. She was aware of these cues though and managed to talk herself out of drinking, if it was not the right time or place – an appropriate response.

Behavioral and cognitive tips are in order if you are tempted by the sight and smell of your preferred cocktail. First, store liquor away from your living area. If you stare at bottles of wine, beer or distilled spirits every time you pass the wine rack, open the refrigerator door or the kitchen cupboard, remove the booze and keep it somewhere else. Just getting it out of your face will reduce the frequency of your craving.

Or desensitize yourself to the sight and smell of liquor. Pick up your drink of choice. Sniff it. Hold it for several minutes and examine it carefully. Then put it down without sipping it. Practice this four or five times in a row without drinking. Hopefully, the powerful impact of the sensory cues associated with your favorite drink which trigger your drinking desire will fade.

And if people drinking in your presence awaken your need for alcohol, talk yourself out of it like Cassie does. Question if it's the right time or place for drinking.

You will crave less and you will drink less if you are aware of what cues trip your drinking desire.

Drinking Places

Imagine you're at your favorite watering hole. A restaurant or club? A friend's house or your home? A social or sporting event? Just being in this special place sets off an alcohol craving in you. Where are your favorite drinking places?

Asa is a great cook and has worked in the restaurant business for years. Alcohol and drinking are occupational hazards for him. It seems everyone he works with drinks heavily. Some drink on the job, which is not allowed but happens anyway. And most nights after closing the restaurant, everyone downs a couple of cocktails and continues partying at the nearest bar. Unfortunately for Asa, his workplace is one big drinking cue. A hazard to his health he thought.

Unhappy with how much he was drinking, he decided to change his ways. For starters, he would stick to business only – not drinking. No more drinking on the job. At the end of his workday he would allow himself two drinks, opt out of the drinking party at the bar and go straight home instead. He not only altered his working and drinking habits, he altered his attitude too. Just recognizing his place of employment was a problem-drinking trap put him on his guard and that insight also helped him to cut down.

Avoid or limit the time you spend at your preferred drinking spot to tame this drinking cue. If you drink at home, get busy and fill the old drinking time with activities that take your mind off of alcohol. And understand that a specific location can lead to alcohol craving and abuse – making you more mindful of and less susceptible to this trigger. Simple solutions to manage a simple cue.

Drinking Companions

Here comes trouble. You just ran into one of your boozing buddies who always wants to drink. His company automatically sets off a drinking response in you and you drink too much when you're with him.

Take another look at Asa. The restaurant was not the only cue that encouraged his heavy drinking. His co-workers were also part of the problem. Ultimately, he not only limited his time at the restaurant, but the time he spent with his pals too. Especially after work.

Avoid or limit the time you spend with people that keep you focused on alcohol. If this is impossible, confide in your friends about your concern over the heavy drinking that takes place when you are in their company. Then suggest cutting down so this will no longer be an issue. If this doesn't work, you may be forced to cut all ties with them. The less time you spend with alcohol abusers, the less time you will abuse alcohol.

Physiological Cues

Hunger

Hunger is one of the most intense human needs known to man and may spark alcohol craving. Some drinkers ignore or misinterpret hunger and drink alcohol instead of eating – a dangerous, inappropriate reaction that could initiate problem drinking.

Drinking on an empty stomach when you're hungry is a bad idea in more ways than one. Alcohol is hard on the stomach lining and gastrointestinal system. It goes to your head, your blood alcohol concentration levels soar and your judgment and decision-making abilities become impaired. Then you lose control, drink more than you should and become a danger to yourself and others – especially if you get behind the wheel of a car. And you end up nursing a nasty hangover the next morning.

Amazing Commonsense Tips to Curb Drinking Desire

Carol is a very busy professional woman who had a drinking problem. She works ten to twelve hours a day, then goes to the gym and gets home at eight or nine at night. Even though she is famished by the end of the day, instead of eating dinner she would collapse on the sofa with a drink. She was too tired to cook and rationalized scotch and water was less fattening than food anyway. Carol's hectic lifestyle also entered into the picture. She looked forward to that first drink because it took the edge off of a stressful day, put her in a good mood and energized her. Unfortunately, the downside to her drinking pattern was feeling slow the next morning. Luckily, Carol realized she was drinking her dinner and if she didn't watch it, she could become an alcoholic. That's when she decided to turn over a new leaf and clean up her drinking act.

She started by recognizing her hunger, not stuffing it, and eating a hearty breakfast and lunch to stabilize her blood sugar levels during the day. On her way home from the gym, she would drink her favorite non-alcoholic beverage – cranberry juice. This healthy drink – loaded with vitamin C and light on calories – took the edge off her hunger and gave her that needed blast of energy. And when she got home she would have a snack – whole wheat crackers. The juice and snack curbed her appetite enabling her to sip, not gulp, that first scotch while making dinner. She enjoyed a second scotch with dinner but had no desire to continue drinking after eating. She felt satisfied.

Carol was surprised at how easy it was to break her old drinking routine. Regular meals, non-alcoholic beverages and snacking kept her hunger at bay, revitalized her and decreased her need for alcohol. She was no longer drinking too fast, going overboard or suffering from "slow hangovers." Or feeling guilty about a growing drinking habit and gaining weight – even though she was eating more food, she was consuming a lot fewer empty scotch calories.

Do you drink alcohol instead of eating when you're hungry? If you's time you recognize your appetite is for food, not liquor – then eat! Next, enjoy a big breakfast and lunch to stabilize your blood sugar levels. When your blood sugar levels are stable, you feel better physically and mentally and you'll find it easier to slow down and pace your drinking. Third, always snack before and during drinking so alcohol doesn't go to your head. Finally, toss that "drinking is less fattening than eating" diet myth out the window – it's not true. These tips could slash your need to drink. No more excuses!

Thirst

Or perhaps thirst gets you started? Another basic human need which must be quenched for survival. Conventional wisdom says you should drink at least eight eight-ounce glasses of water every day. Most of us don't come close to that and only drink water when we are parched. The problem is some people drink alcohol in place of water to satisfy thirst. Another inappropriate response that could lead to alcohol abuse.

Ed is a construction worker. During the warm weather months, he works twelve hour days. And even though other physiological factors played a role in his desire to drink, thirst was a major drinking cue for him. After a long, hot day, the first thing on his mind was an ice cold beer. He was up to six beers a day and often bypassed eating in favor of drinking. Concerned he was on the road to alcoholism, he sought help.

Now, instead of starting the evening with a beer after a hard day's work, Ed's new routine starts with ice water. It takes care of his thirst and his craving for beer. Then he enjoys a beer or two and dinner and doesn't feel the need to continue drinking. Discovering the thirst variable and satisfying it logically made cutting down on alcohol simple for him.

Does thirst enter into your drinking picture? Drinking plenty of fluids during the day and before you start drinking may make a world of difference in your alcohol consumption too.

Fatigue

Do you turn to alcohol for energy? Especially in the late afternoon or early evening when you are starting to fade? Confusing the need to revitalize yourself with the need to drink is a big mistake for some people.

Elliot is a computer executive who works a lot and is a good example of the "rest" cure for alcohol craving. Several days a week, instead of commuting to work in his car, he takes the bus. He noticed he drank less on his "bus" days and thought the catnap he took on the ride home was responsible for his cutting down. After snoozing on the bus, he felt refreshed, relaxed and not nearly as interested in a martini when he got home.

Elliot then realized when he felt tired and needed a lift he looked to alcohol to recharge his batteries. And on the flip side, if he took a rest break his desire to drink diminished. He decided taking the bus was a smart move in more ways than one – it reduced his stress level, increased his energy level and decreased his alcohol appetite.

Instead of relying on an early cocktail hour to perk yourself up, take a break. Grab a catnap in the afternoon. Or treat yourself to "tea time" – refreshments to elevate your blood sugar levels and mood – around three or four. You'll feel refreshed and energized and not nearly as vulnerable to alcohol craving. Rest up and watch alcohol consumption go down!

Sleeping Aid

Is alcohol your sleeping pill at night? If it is, it shouldn't be and it's up to you to explore other options so you get your rest without it.

Lisa knows drinking to fall asleep is unacceptable, but a hard habit to break. She is "on" all day and has a hard time turning "off" at night. Lisa has no problem limiting herself to two cocktails with dinner, but when eleven rolls around and she is still "on" she will have two more to put herself out. She rationalizes if she doesn't drink at bedtime she'll never get to sleep and be a zombie at work the next day. So, instead of tossing and turning for hours, she gives in to the nightcaps. But those extra drinks just before bed took their toll on her the next morning. That's when she decided to cut out bedtime drinking.

Here's what Lisa did so getting to sleep was no longer an excuse to drink. First, she studied up on healthy sleeping habits, looked at her current night-time pattern and brainstormed ways she could improve it without alcohol. In place of an extra drink, perhaps she would have an herbal tea or soak in a hot bath before she retired. TV or reading in bed was not allowed – unless it put her to sleep. She also thought about listening to a relaxation tape or practicing her favorite relaxation exercises. If all else failed, she decided she would talk to her doctor about the problem. Maybe sleeping medication would be the answer. But relaxing with a bubble bath and sipping a calming tea before bed did it for Lisa. She succeeded in getting a good night's rest without alcohol and cut her drinking in half.

If you rely on liquor to get to sleep keep in mind too much alcohol actually disrupts sleep. It causes restless sleep. And you wake up in the morning feeling groggy and hungover from too much alcohol and too little sleep. If you stay within your drink limit, however, you should sleep like a baby and feel great the next day. Two of many rewards for sticking to moderate drinking.

Pain or Physical Discomfort

When was the last time you prescribed a drink for yourself? If you suffer from a painful medical or dental condition, if you have a physically demanding job or if you are challenged with the aches and pains of just getting older, you may be familiar with this type of problem drinking. And medicating yourself with alcohol is not the answer.

Remember Ed? The construction worker whose thirst played into his desire to drink? Relieving sprains, bumps and bruises with booze was another factor that caused him to drink too much. If he was hurting at the end of the day, instead of popping an aspirin, soaking in a hot tub or getting a massage to feel better, he would reach for a beer. Fortunately, he also recognized this drinking cue and started dealing with it appropriately.

Sam was in his 70's, didn't have a lot to occupy his time and didn't get out much because of arthritis pain. Once he determined that boredom and physical discomfort were the culprits behind his drinking problem, he set out to make things right. He saw his doctor, got medication and started an exercise routine to manage his arthritis while pursuing new interests. Drinking less alcohol was his payoff for dealing with the situation proactively.

Time to get real if you treat yourself with alcohol. Take a good look at this nasty little habit, use a little commonsense and start addressing physiological needs sensibly. Take a pain reliever, get out the heating pad or go to the physical therapist to feel better. See your doctor or dentist about a medical or dental condition. Baby boomers and seniors – you know the aging process is no picnic. Arthritis, rheumatism, and other ailments go with the territory and should be treated by a professional.

Assume responsibility for feeling good physically and watch your need to drink evaporate.

Psychological Cues

Emotions

Is alcohol your therapist? Do you drink too much to soothe negative feelings – anger, frustration or loneliness? Or do you drink too much to enhance positive feelings – to toast good times or reward yourself? Sharpening your emotional awareness and realizing you may be overdrinking in response to feelings may help to deflate your alcohol craving.

Cindy knows celebrating too much of nothing gives her a hangover the next day. Any excuse for a party and she will give herself permission to get smashed. Whenever Les makes a sale he has to paint the town. Getting drunk three or four times a month is not unusual. If one of Rod's real estate transactions falls through, he will tie one on and drown his frustration in liquor. Kathy drinks too much when she gets angry. If anything gets her goat, she binges. May is a senior citizen with nothing to do. Bored and lonely, she drinks to fill the time.

If things are going your way, enjoy yourself with one or two cocktails – sensible, moderate drinking. If things are not going your way, try a more thoughtful approach than alcohol. First, tune in to the emotions you are feeling – don't mask them with booze. Second, examine the issues behind the emotions. Next, analyze different solutions to resolve these issues so they don't stir negative feelings. Then follow through with the best solution. Also, learn to cope with your emotions in a healthier way –

talk about them, write about them, let off steam with a run, treat yourself to chocolate, beat a pillow – whatever works for you.

If increasing your emotional awareness, self-help and coping methods don't do the trick, look into professional counseling. Do emotions spark your drinking desire?

Moods and States of Mind

Does anxiety, depression or stress drive you to drink? Research shows these moods and states of mind are common drinking triggers. And the bad news is treating these moods with alcohol often aggravates them, prevents you from addressing them and leads to even more problem drinking.

Deena had suffered from clinical depression for years. She had also been drinking heavily for years and her alcohol consumption was on the rise. Wine gave her a break from the blues she struggled with most days. Bridget experienced panic attacks. But instead of seeing a counselor for the problem, she drank. And Steven worked at least eighty hours a week subsisting on junk food, no exercise and little sleep. He was stressed physiologically and psychologically and vodka simply made him feel better fast.

If you suffer from anxiety, depression or stress and drink alcohol to improve your mood, you need help. Go to the library, study up on what's troubling you and check out proven mood-elevating and stress-reducing strategies and techniques. For example, schedule at least one "free" day a week to play – free from business or household chores. Or exercise for an endorphin rush and to increase feelings of well-being. Plan and follow through with activities you enjoy to take your mind off of what's eating you. Laugh. Organize and prioritize daily tasks so you get the most important chores done and save the rest for another day. Listen to music. Cultivate a "nothing is the end of the world" attitude. Eat pasta. Be good to yourself and splurge on your favorite cologne or share a fine bottle of wine with good friends. Do something special every week – a trip to the country or a concert? Relax at a spa. Take up meditation, prayer or mental relaxation exercises. Plan a quiet time every day to collect your thoughts and re-energize. Take short breaks often during the workday. Talk issues out with people you trust.

Perhaps looking into a support group in your area to help you deal with the problem at hand would be helpful. Or professional counseling might do you good. Contact your local non-profit mental health agency for assistance. A counselor may be able to help you live the life you deserve without alcohol abuse.

Relieving psychological pain can relieve alcohol craving. How often is your desire to drink linked to your mood?

Beliefs and Expectations

Deep down inside each one of us, we hold certain beliefs and expectations about alcohol and drinking we learned from parents and peers. Alcohol is good or bad. Alcohol is a social lubricant. Alcohol makes you smarter and sexier. Drinking alcohol is a must to part of the "in" crowd. Bingeing and getting drunk is OK every once in a while. What are your deep-seated beliefs and expectations about drinking and alcohol?

Brendan started bingeing in his early teens. He never outgrew it and this behavior continued into his thirties. Brendan looked at booze in black and white terms. You were "good" if you did not drink at all. But if you did drink, you were "bad" so you might as well go all out and get drunk. One odd set of beliefs about drinking and alcohol.

Sally thought she was a big hit when she had one too many. After a couple of gin and tonics she felt more confident, would do things she would not ordinarily do and thought she was the life of the party. When she was tipsy, she got plenty of attention – especially from the opposite sex. And even though her drunken escapades got her into trouble occasionally, she only remembers the good times. She thinks of how funny, sexy and sassy she feels when she gets to drink number four. Of course, the next day she pays for these misconceptions with a hangover and lots of gossip about her out-of-control drinking. Time for an attitude adjustment, Sally.

Now, let's separate fact from fiction about alcohol and drinking. Alcohol is not good or bad. How you use alcohol determines its worth. A few drinks may enhance your social and sex life, but too much booze could make you obnoxious and impotent. One or two drinks could make you sharper mentally, but too many will turn you into a zombie. And if liquor is required to be accepted by the "in" crowd, you're hanging out with the wrong crowd – people who value alcohol way too much. Bingeing and getting smashed are never OK. And just because you have a couple of drinks does not mean you have to go overboard and get drunk. Drinking alcohol in moderation is adult behavior and can improve the quality of your life. It should be the goal of any drinker.

Correcting misconceptions you have about alcohol may decrease your need to drink. Is it time for your attitude adjustment?

Even More Amazing Anti-Craving, Moderate Drinking Tips . . .

No More Cigarettes

Canadian scientists have found that nicotine in cigarettes increases the urge to drink alcohol. They think there is a biological process common to the use and abuse of both alcohol and tobacco. They also think that nicotine and alcohol share the same reward process in the brain. If you smoke, quit. If you don't smoke, don't start!

Fine Tune Your Attitude to Manage Craving

Keeping your head and a positive, confident attitude when you are faced with a strong alcohol craving is a must to beating it. Who's in charge? You or your craving? You are! Bigger and stronger than any desire to drink!

It's also important you accept craving as a normal part of the changing process if you are cutting down on your alcohol consumption. In the beginning, cravings will be intense in high-risk situations but will fade over time, if you practice your anti-craving strategies and skills to defuse them.

Delay

Psychologists say if you delay drinking for ten or fifteen minutes there is a good chance your craving will pass. Think of it. Just with the passage of time you can douse your drinking desire!

From now on, when the urge strikes, look at your watch and give yourself a ten-minute timeout before giving into it. And notice the desire has diminished or passed when the time's up. This patient approach has been proven to reduce alcohol consumption.

Distract

Next time the need to drink gets the better of you, distract yourself with activities that don't involve alcohol to keep your appetite at bay. Pet the dog, brush your teeth, have a snack. Practice deep breathing and relaxation exercises. Anything to get your mind off of alcohol and craving.

Express Yourself

On the other hand, focusing on your miserable craving might do the trick. Call a friend and talk to them about your feelings when you're wrestling with a strong drinking desire. Or start a craving journal and record your thoughts and feelings when you are suffering from a red-hot urge. You'll be killing three birds with one stone – you'll be heightening your craving awareness, you'll be getting your feelings about the painful craving experience off your chest and you'll be decreasing your desire to drink all at the same time.

Step on Your Craving with Basic Moderate Drinking Tools

Research shows if you pre-plan drinking behavior with basic moderate drinking strategies and techniques, the more successful you will be at reducing your alcohol craving and consumption.

Next time you're faced with a drinking challenge, before you even start drinking, plan on how long you'll drink, how many drinks you'll have and how long you'll nurse each drink. Rehearse the plan in your head and saying "no" to another drink which may put you over your limit. Knowing when to stop drinking before you even start may cut your drinking desire and alcohol intake.

For more moderate drinking tools pick up the book, *7 Weeks to Safe Social Drinking: How to Effectively Moderate Your Alcohol Intake,* by Donna J. Cornett.

Forget the Guilt and Remember Why You Want to Cut Down

If you slip off the moderate-drinking track, don't wallow in guilt or shame. These negative feelings are counterproductive and might lead to even more drinking. Instead, get back on track immediately and remind yourself of all the reasons why you want to beat craving and problem drinking. And remember how you will transform your life if you stick with safe, social drinking. It's a brand new day!

The Craving Game

What drinking cues push your buttons? Record the internal and external cues that trigger your alcohol appetite in your Craving Diary. Internal cues, like hunger, thirst, fatigue and pain and mood cues, like joy, satisfaction, anger, frustration, anxiety, stress and depression. External cues, including the time of day, the company you keep and the location where the urge strikes. Then devote time and energy to dealing with these cues appropriately so they don't get in the way of your moderate drinking goal.

Part Three:
WESTERN APPROACHES
TO BEAT ALCOHOL CRAVING

Chapter 6

Outsmart the Drinking Urge with Nutritional Supplements

Restoring nutritional deficiencies and supplementing your diet with specific vitamins, minerals and amino acids may be the keys to reducing alcohol craving and consumption, according to some nutritionists. This chapter digs into dietary supplements to correct shortages, purify the body, and stabilize the mood so you eliminate the physiological and psychological see-saw that produces alcohol craving and drives you to drink.

Some experts believe more than fifty percent of alcoholics suffer from nutritional deficiencies and imbalances. The late Dr. Robert Atkins claimed thirty to thirty-five percent of alcoholics may be able to quit drinking with the help of therapy and AA alone. But with nutritional supplementation, in addition to therapy and AA, expect seventy-five to eighty percent of alcoholics to successfully abstain, according to Atkins.

What causes nutritional deficiencies? Chronic heavy drinking and poor eating habits. Alcohol breaks down in the liver and long-term alcohol abuse inhibits the production of digestive enzymes in the liver, so the body is unable to absorb fat and protein. Important vitamins, like A, B, C, D and E, and minerals, including magnesium, selenium and zinc, also become difficult to absorb and are eliminated through urine. Plus, alcohol is full of empty calories with no nutritional value. So when you slip into bad eating habits and drink your dinner, you don't get the vitamins you need. However, if you cut down on your drinking, eat a well-balanced diet and take a megavitamin, you should be able to reverse this malabsorption and retain nutrients so you feel better in no time.

Heavy drinking not only causes vitamin shortages, it also produces acetaldehyde – the villain of alcohol use. This toxic chemical is produced in the body when you metabolize alcohol. Too much alcohol increases acetaldehyde and free radical formation – free radicals are dangerous substances that cause cell damage and disease. Acetaldehyde and free radicals cause a number of health problems, including cancer, liver and heart disease, premature aging and a weakened immune system. Extra supplements to rid the body of alcohol-related toxins and reduce the harmful effects of acetaldehyde are also on the agenda.

The "Daily Value" of a supplement is the average daily intake of a nutrient that meets the requirements of most healthy people, according to the U.S. Food and Drug Administration Center for Food Safety and Applied Nutrition. The Daily Value for each vitamin and mineral is listed, but the agency has not yet established a Daily Value for amino acids so none are listed. Amino acid supplements are recommended because only trace amounts of many amino acids are found in foods.

It seems there are as many different nutritional approaches to treat alcohol abuse as there are nutritionists. Here we have pinned down the dietary aids common to many programs and thought to be the most effective. Some of these supplements may function in several different ways, but will be listed in only one category. For example, versatile niacin and GABA may not only calm the nerves, but they may also reduce the desire to drink. Just a reminder – the nutrients are listed in alphabetical order in each section, not in the order of their importance.

You must seek the advice of your physician if you consider any one of these supplements. The wrong supplement or dosage may be hazardous to your health, interact with over-the-counter and prescription medications or exacerbate a pre-existing medical or psychological condition.

First, Restore Deficiencies and
Get Rid of Alcohol-Related Toxins

Multivitamin and Mineral Supplement

Start by covering all of your bases with a well-balanced diet – covered in Chapter Four – and a megavitamin and mineral supplement. This easy first step helps one to retain and absorb vitamins, minerals, fatty acids, enzymes and amino acids essential for good health, a positive attitude and decreased drinking desire.

Vitamin A

Vitamin A, also known as retinol, is needed for healthy skin, hair, teeth and gums. It plays an important role in cell division and differentiation, bone growth, eyesight and reproduction. The U.S. Food and Drug Administration Center for Food Safety and Applied Nutrition states vitamin A is required for a strong immune system.

An A deficiency is common in alcohol abusers – the vitamin is excreted in bile during the alcohol metabolism process. If you are lacking in vitamin A, you may suffer from dry skin, diarrhea, night blindness, kidney stones, eye disease and respiratory infections.

Adding A to the diet is recommended to prevent liver disease, cure night blindness and correct sexual problems. Plus, drinkers short on A show improved taste and smell when supplemented with the vitamin.

The Daily Value for vitamin A is 5,000 international units. Natural food sources of A include leafy greens, yams, sweet potatoes, vegetables, fruits, eggs and liver. Most fat-free and dried nonfat milk and many breakfast cereals are fortified with A.

Be careful – too much vitamin A could damage the liver. Do not drink heavily if you take extra A because it could speed the development of liver disease. Taking too much of the vitamin may be dangerous and result in vomiting, hair loss, osteoporosis, blurred vision and vision problems. Pregnant and breastfeeding women should avoid A since it can cause birth defects. Consult a nutritionist or nutritionally-aware physician before you get serious about vitamin A.

Vitamin B Complex

B-complex vitamins are required for many body functions and heavy drinkers often suffer from B shortages. Beautiful B's cleanse the body, improve the mood and tame the urge to drink. They provide varied results when taken individually, so ideally they should be taken together in a B-complex supplement for the best results.

Vitamin B1

Vitamin B1 or thiamin is a tonic for the body and soul. It promotes healthy circulation, digestion, metabolism and nerve transmission, it contributes to growth and physical development and it is necessary for converting carbohydrates into energy in the muscle and nervous systems. An antioxidant, it removes poisonous alcohol by-products from the body and protects it from the effects of alcohol, nicotine and aging. The U.S.

Food and Drug Administration believes the vitamin is necessary for a healthy nervous system.

A vitamin B1 deficiency is the most common deficiency among alcohol abusers. Depression, irritability, insomnia, indigestion, poor muscle coordination, edema, heart failure and beriberi are all symptoms of a B1 shortage. It may also cause psychiatric and neurological problems, increased alcohol consumption and alcohol abuse.

Vitamin B1 is also known as the "morale" vitamin because of its positive psychological effects. Extra B1 may relieve depression – a major factor contributing to alcohol craving and problem drinking for some people. It improves appetite and mental acuity and it is used to treat learning problems, emotional disorders, Alzheimer's disease, motion sickness and fatigue. B1 boosts the immune system.

Animal studies by Eriksson, Pekkanen and Rusi indicate supplemental thiamin may also reduce drinking. In one study, rats were fed diets containing different amounts of thiamin. Rats on a thiamin-deficient diet showed a significant tendency towards increased alcohol consumption compared to rats on a diet containing thiamin.

The Daily Value for thiamin is 1.5 milligrams. Vitamin B1 can be found naturally in beef liver, kidney, ham, dried garbanzo beans, kidney beans, navy beans, raw brown rice, wheat germ, oranges, flour, rye, and whole grain products.

No problems have been reported with taking large doses of B1 over a long period of time.

Vitamin B2

Vitamin B2 or riboflavin is another mind/body miracle. It is needed to make red blood cells and antibodies and for cell growth, to maintain skin and eye tissues and to metabolize other B vitamins. Along with vitamin A, it keeps the digestive tract healthy and utilizes proteins, carbohydrates, fatty acids and amino acids. Riboflavin is also needed to produce glutathione – a powerful antioxidant.

Heavy drinkers often lack B2. A deficiency impairs iron absorption in the body, weakens the thyroid gland and contributes to depression and mental health problems. Skin conditions, hair loss, indigestion, sores around the corners of the mouth, eye disease and a lack of mental focus are also associated with a vitamin B2 shortage.

Glutathione, the antioxidant powerhouse which riboflavin helps produce, prevents disease and slows the aging process. It detoxifies and improves liver function, aids vision in general, prevents cataracts and fortifies the immune system. This super antioxidant is the accepted treatment for liver failure caused by acetaminophen poisoning and it is also given for respiratory problems, hair loss, sickle cell anemia, psoriasis and cell damage caused by stroke or heart attack. Take your vitamin B2 and get a glutathione bonus! Low levels of glutathione have been linked to cancer, heart disease, arthritis and diabetes.

The Daily Value of riboflavin is 1.7 milligrams. Whole grains, meat, fish, poultry, nuts and eggs are good sources of vitamin B2. Cheese, asparagus, broccoli and mushrooms also contain the vitamin.

No problems have been reported with taking large doses of vitamin B2 over a long period of time.

Vitamin C

Vitamin C is truly a multipurpose vitamin which chases away disease and maintains good health. According to the U.S. Food and Drug Administration Center for Food Safety and Applied Nutrition, it is vital for healthy skin, bones and teeth, it activates liver-detoxifying systems in the body and it protects you from cancer-causing carcinogens. C is required to make collagen – connective tissue protein necessary for tissue growth and repair – and to metabolize amino acids and hormones needed for normal adrenal gland functioning.

Unfortunately, research shows heavy drinkers are often lacking in antioxidants, including vitamin C. In fact, studies have shown a correlation between antioxidants, free radical levels and liver damage from alcohol abuse: the greater the antioxidant deficiency, the greater the liver damage. Other symptoms of a C shortage include digestive problems, increased infections, low energy, bleeding gums and easy bruising.

Vitamin C possesses antibacterial, anti-inflammatory and anti-cancer properties. It scavenges free radicals and fights off infections, viruses, allergies, asthma, gallstones, cancer, heart disease and stress. The vitamin reduces high blood pressure and cholesterol levels, prevents arteriosclerosis and enhances the immune system.

Mighty C has been shown to reduce toxin levels in the liver and body. And it actually speeds the clearance of alcohol from the blood stream. Taking vitamin C before, during or after drinking prevents fatty deposits in the liver (the first sign of liver disease) caused by too much alcohol.

The Daily Value of vitamin C is 60 milligrams. If supplements are not for you, eat dark green vegetables, including broccoli, brussel sprouts, kale, parsley, cabbage, collard and turnip greens – all rich in the vitamin. Citrus fruits, mangoes, guavas, strawberries, papaya, tomatoes and melons are also excellent C sources.

More than 1,000 milligrams of vitamin C a day may cause an upset stomach and diarrhea. Large doses of vitamin C are not recommended for individuals with kidney problems or genetic conditions that lead to iron overload.

Vitamin E

Another awesome antioxidant which combats free radicals and the harmful effects of alcohol, vitamin E is needed to maintain nerves, muscles, skin, hair and eyes and is required for tissue repair and blood clotting. It has earned the reputation of being a cancer, heart disease, diabetes, arthritis, menopause and cataract fighter. Where would you be without your vitamin E?

Even though a vitamin E deficiency is rare, a drinker may reap the benefits of extra E. According to the U.S. Food and Drug Administration, the vitamin not only detoxifies free radicals and prevents cell membrane damage, it also prevents early-stage liver disease from progressing and arterial plaque buildup which may lead to heart disease. It's a real immune system booster too.

Animal studies have shown alcohol reduces E in liver cells. Human studies have shown too much alcohol reduces E in the heart muscle. And like vitamin C, taking E before, during or after drinking may inhibit the development of fatty deposits in the liver and prevent liver disease.

The Daily Value of vitamin E is 30 international units. Spinach, dandelion, mustard and turnip greens, kale, wheat germ, peanuts, almonds, margarine, soybean and sunflower oils are all rich in the vitamin. Eggs, brown rice and oatmeal are also good sources of E.

Caution should be taken with vitamin E. High doses of E interfere with other fat-soluble vitamins – especially vitamin K. If you are interested in extra E, consult your physician, particularly if you take anticoagulants or aspirin regularly, have high blood pressure, heart disease or cancer.

Magnesium

This incredible mineral activates more than 100 enzymes and is crucial for over 300 biological processes in the body! Magnesium is essential for bone growth and nerve and muscle functioning – including regulating normal heart rhythm. It also works as an antacid and laxative and strengthens tooth enamel. Magnesium is given to treat heart and kidney disease, high blood pressure, blood sugar disorders, asthma, migraines and osteoporosis.

Alcohol abuse depletes magnesium in the body. It is estimated thirty to sixty percent of alcoholics suffer from a magnesium deficiency. Alcohol increases the elimination of the mineral in urine causing a shortage which can lead to depression, confusion, loss of appetite, muscle cramps, irregular heartbeat and seizures. Not getting enough of the mineral can also cause heart and muscle disease. That's the bad news. The good news is many of these conditions can be corrected immediately with a little magnesium.

The mineral is not only a blessing for the body, it's great for the spirit too. It is known as the "anti-anxiety" mineral and is used to calm mild anxiety and promote restful sleep.

The Daily Value is 400 milligrams. Natural sources include avocados, dairy products, halibut, herring, leafy green vegetables, nuts, wheat germ and whole wheat bread.

Too much magnesium may cause diarrhea, nausea, muscle weakness, low blood pressure, breathing difficulty and irregular heart beat. It could be fatal for people with kidney disease. If you suffer from heart or kidney disease, low blood pressure or migraine headaches talk to your nutritionally-aware physician about this mineral.

Selenium

Selenium is a must to get rid of dangerous alcohol by-products in the body. This mineral prevents free radical formation and damage and is necessary for normal growth and development. Together with vitamin E, it produces antibodies which maintain a healthy heart and liver. This anti-inflammatory, anti-cancer antioxidant is prescribed for heart disease, cancer, arthritis, pancreatitis, thyroid disease and AIDS. It also enhances the immune system.

The U.S. Food and Drug Administration recognizes selenium as a potent alcohol detoxifier. It has liver-protecting properties, especially for people suffering from cirrhosis caused by heavy drinking. Specifically, selenium activates glutathione peroxidase, an enzyme which protects the liver from damage caused by alcohol abuse. When you are short on selenium, you are short on this liver-protecting enzyme too. A selenium deficiency is not only associated with liver disease, it also leads to heart disease and alcoholic myopathy, an illness affecting the major muscle groups of the body.

The Daily Value of selenium is 70 micrograms. Feast on dairy products, chicken, liver, whole grains, Brazil nuts, garlic and wheat germ as alternatives to supplements. Salmon, tuna, brown rice and broccoli are also loaded with the mineral.

Large doses of selenium are dangerous. More than 200 micrograms of selenium may cause stomach upset, diarrhea, fatigue, irritability, numbness in the extremities and changes in hair, nails and mental functioning. The mineral may mutate cells and cause cancer. See your doctor or nutritionist if you are considering selenium supplementation.

Zinc

Zinc is required for the functioning of every cell in your body. It promotes normal growth and development and keeps your senses of taste and smell in tact. This mineral is the source of many important enzymes and prevents free radical formation. It is a healing agent and a mood and immune system booster. Zinc is given for colds, acne, cancer and infertility.

A zinc deficiency has been observed in thirty to fifty percent of alcoholics. Excessive alcohol consumption increases zinc lost in urine and decreases the absorption of the mineral in the body. Not enough zinc may lead to psychiatric disorders, heart, brain and nervous system diseases, indigestion, allergies, poor wound healing, fatigue, colds, skin problems and more!

A zinc shortage can also lead to liver disease. It is a key nutrient in the breakdown of alcohol and guards the liver from chemical damage. Specifically, aldehyde dehydrogenase, the enzyme which renders acetaldehyde harmless, requires zinc to be effective. Remember – acetaldehyde is the toxic by-product of alcohol metabolism. If zinc levels are low, aldehyde dehydrogenase activity decreases and may result in liver disease. But when zinc is restored, aldehyde dehydrogenase activity increases and acetaldehyde decreases – reducing the risk of liver problems. Pairing zinc with vitamin C has been shown to increase alcohol detoxification in rats.

The Daily Value of zinc is 15 milligrams. Oysters contain more zinc than any other food, although poultry and red meat provide most of the zinc we need. Pork, yogurt, cashews and fortified breakfast cereals are also good sources of the mineral.

Taking too much zinc may result in deficiencies of other minerals, like iron, copper and manganese, and cause anemia. It may also cause gastrointestinal upset, weight gain and a weakened immune system. Overdosing on zinc over a long period depresses HDL "good" cholesterol. Consult your physician if you are thinking of zincing.

Next, Stabilize Your Mood

Vitamin B12

Another beautiful B vitamin! Also known as cobalamin, B12 keeps your nerve and red blood cells healthy, plays a big part in DNA production, improves concentration and strengthens the immune system. It has anti-inflammatory and pain-relieving qualities and is recommended to relieve hangovers, depression and fatigue and to lift the spirits.

When one suffers from a vitamin B12 deficiency, mood disturbances, including depression, may occur. And feeling blue is one powerful drinking cue for many people. Confusion, poor memory, fatigue, anemia, dizziness and nervous system, neurological and heart problems are also symptoms of a B12 shortage. Oral contraceptives, cholesterol, anti-inflammatory and anti-convulsive medications may deplete this vitamin.

Even if you are not lacking in B12, research suggests adding it to your diet may improve your mood. And a positive outlook could translate into decreased drinking desire.

The Daily Value of vitamin B12 is 6 micrograms. Food sources of the vitamin include poultry, meat, organ meats, fish, eggs, cheese, milk and fortified breakfast cereals.

There are no problems reported with high doses of vitamin B12.

Calcium

Calcium is famous for its calming effect, in addition to being a strong bone and tooth builder. It is essential for normal growth and development and it helps to regulate heartbeat, blood clotting and muscle contractions. The mineral may lower blood pressure and cholesterol levels and prevent cancer and osteoporosis. It is also involved in energy production and fortifies the immune system. A shortage causes brittle bones, muscle spasms, irregular heartbeat, aching joints, dementia, insomnia and depression.

The U.S. Food and Drug Administration Center for Food Safety and Applied Nutrition reports anecdotal evidence supports the use of calcium as a tranquilizer. It soothes anxiety and promotes restful sleep and the more relaxed and well-rested you feel, the less you need alcohol.

The Daily Value of calcium is 1,000 milligrams. If you are not into supplements or dairy products loaded with calcium, sardines, salmon with bones, almonds, sesame seeds, Brazil nuts, spinach, kale, swiss chard and pinto beans are good alternatives.

Too much calcium in the diet may cause kidney disease, constipation, tissue calcification and a magnesium shortage. If you have kidney problems, check with your doctor before taking calcium.

GABA

Often referred to as the body's natural tranquilizer, gamma-aminobutyric acid or GABA is an amino acid that may keep you cool, calm and collected – and might even reduce your alcohol craving.

Amino acids help you to metabolize vitamins and minerals and are the building blocks of neurotransmitters. Neurotransmitters are powerful brain chemicals linked to mood, craving and addictive behavior. Restoring specific amino acids will restore neurotransmitters which may elevate mood and douse the desire to drink.

Considered a safe nutritional tranquilizer, GABA prevents anxiety and stress messages from reaching the brain. It brings on relaxation and restful sleep, but is not addictive. This amino acid is given for anxiety, depression, panic attacks, convulsions, epilepsy, hypertension, PMS and attention deficit disorder.

No Daily Value has been established for GABA. Vegetable and animal protein, along with other vitamins and minerals, are the precursors of GABA production.

Nausea, anxiety and shortness of breath may result from taking too much GABA. It may interact with other medications. See your nutritionist or physician before you experiment with GABA.

L-Methionine

The amino acid supplement of methionine, L-methionine has been prescribed by psychiatrists to relieve depression for decades. Fatty liver, slow growth, edema, skin problems and dementia are all symptoms of a methionine deficiency.

L-methionine is a central nervous system depressant and improves the attitude of people coping with moderate to major depression. The amino acid is also a strong antioxidant which inactivates free radicals and prevents and breaks down fatty buildup in the liver and arteries which may limit blood flow to the heart, brain and kidneys. Research shows it aids digestion, detoxifies the liver and effectively treats cirrhosis and hepatitis. It not only alleviates depression and improves liver function, some think it reduces alcohol craving too. The perfect combination for a drinker!

Individuals suffering from pancreatitis, Parkinson's disease, schizophrenia and HIV/AIDS may benefit from extra L-methionine.

Osteoarthritis, chronic fatigue syndrome and neurological disorders are also treated with the amino acid.

A Daily Value has not been established for methionine. Food sources include meat, fish, eggs, soybeans, yogurt, onions and garlic.

Little information is available on the side effects of L-methionine. However, some studies suggest it might affect short-term memory. Best to discuss L-methionine with your nutritionally-aware healthcare provider before trying it.

L-Phenylalanine

The supplemental form of the amino acid phenylalanine, L-phenylalanine increases neurotransmitters which alleviate depression and pain, elevate mood, increase pleasure and mental alertness and suppress appetite. Depression, low energy, inability to concentrate, sensitivity to pain, skin and liver problems are symptoms of a phenylalanine shortage.

There are three different types of phenylalanine: L, D and DL. The L-form sharpens memory and mental ability and steps on appetite. The D-form relieves pain. And the DL-form is a combination of the two.

Preliminary studies show L-phenylalanine brightens the outlook of depressed people. In one study, the D and L forms of the amino acid reduced depression in thirty-one of forty people. Another study showed the combined D and L forms relieved depression as well as a prescription antidepressant drug. Claims have been made it curbs sugar and alcohol cravings. Arthritis, migraines, obesity and schizophrenia are also treated with the supplement.

No Daily Value has been established for phenylalanine. Pork, poultry, dairy products, nuts and seeds contain this amino acid.

L-phenylalanine may increase blood pressure and heart rate. Side effects of too much of the supplement include nausea, headache and nerve damage. Do not take this amino acid if you are pregnant, have high blood pressure or if you suffer from anxiety attacks, the genetic disease PKU or melanoma. This supplement may interact with other medications. Consult your nutritionist or doctor before considering L-phenylalanine.

L-Tyrosine

The amino acid supplement of tyrosine, L-tyrosine is considered better than most antidepressant drugs on the market and costs a lot less. It restores dopamine, epinephrine and norepinephrine which are neurotransmitters needed for nerve transmission and to prevent depression. If you are short on tyrosine, you may feel low energy, depressed and unable to focus. Thyroid problems and low blood pressure and body temperature are also symptoms of a deficiency.

Clinical research shows L-tyrosine supplementation not only chases away the blues, it also increases energy and the ability to concentrate and it decreases the need to drink. L-tyrosine is also given for anxiety, stress, headache and fatigue and to aid adrenal, thyroid and pituitary gland functions.

No Daily Value has been established for tyrosine. Dietary sources include dairy products, meat, avocados, bananas, apples, soybeans, carrots, pumpkin and sesame seeds.

L-tyrosine may increase blood pressure and heart rate. Persons taking MAO inhibiters prescribed for depression should limit their use of this supplement. People with a history of skin cancer and high blood pressure should not take this amino acid. Seeing your physician would be a smart move before proceeding with L-tyrosine.

Now, Target Your Drinking Urge

Vitamin B3

Sound the trumpets! Another fabulous B vitamin that purifies the body, lifts the spirits and lessens alcohol craving all rolled into one. Versatile vitamin B3 or niacin promotes good circulation, proper digestion and healthy skin and nerves. It gives you that get up and go feeling – playing a role in cell respiration, fat, protein and carbohydrate metabolism and the release of energy in the body. The vitamin is often given to relieve depression and migraines, improve digestion and reduce the risk of a heart attack.

Many drinkers suffer from a B3 shortage. Not enough niacin can cause depression, fatigue, headache, insomnia, low blood sugar, indigestion, diarrhea, canker sores, skin ailments, loss of appetite and muscle weakness.

Even if a drinker is not lacking in the vitamin they may benefit from adding extra B3 to their diet. Animal and human studies show niacin is an alcohol detoxifier. It interferes with the production of acetaldehyde – the toxic chemical produced by alcohol use which causes liver and heart disease. Improved mood and decreased drinking desire are also associated with more B3 in the diet.

Research shows when drinkers are given niacin or niacinamide, a form of niacin, many enjoy reduced alcohol craving and drink less. In 1974, Dr. Russell Smith successfully treated over 507 alcoholics relying mostly on niacinamide supplementation. Each patient was given a daily dose of the vitamin for five years. The alcoholics relapsed less often and experienced fewer symptoms of alcoholism with the B3 treatment. In 1985, Dr. John Cleary noted some alcoholics spontaneously stopped drinking when given niacin supplements. In another 1990 study, he gave drinkers time-released niacin over a three to four week period. Cleary observed the patients felt less craving, but the craving returned when the niacin was stopped.

The Daily Value for niacin is 20 milligrams. It is found in beef liver, white chicken meat, salmon, tuna, dried beans, green leafy vegetables, peas, potatoes, peanuts and fortified cereals.

Side effects of vitamin B3 may include stomach upset, itching, flushing, dry skin, skin discoloration, peptic ulcer aggravation and hepatitis symptoms. The vitamin is dangerous in high doses. Too much can cause dilation of the blood vessels, a drop in blood pressure, high blood glucose levels and liver disease and failure. If you are allergic to any B vitamin, suffer from liver or kidney disease or if you are pregnant or breastfeeding, consult your healthcare professional before experimenting with vitamin B3.

L-Glutamine

L-glutamine, the supplemental form of the amino acid glutamine, is the most popular nutritional aid to reduce alcohol craving and is routinely given to patients in alcohol abuse treatment clinics across the country. L-glutamine is also credited with relieving stress, enhancing mood and mental alertness and promoting clear thinking. In addition to being an anti-alcohol craving agent, it is often recommended to curb sugar and carbohydrate urges. Depression, fatigue, behavioral problems, schizophrenia, autism, impotence, diabetes and peptic ulcers are all treated with the supplement.

One reason why some scientists believe it defuses the desire to drink is because it elevates and maintains mood. The amino acid is the building block of several neurotransmitters which affect mood and are thought to balance excited and lethargic feelings. Again, the better you feel the less interest you will have in alcohol.

Another reason why some think L-glutamine reduces alcohol craving is because of its ability to stabilize blood sugar levels. If you suffer from low blood sugar, the hypothalamus or appetite center in your brain sends the message to eat foods that will raise your blood sugar levels. In the beginning alcohol accomplishes this, but continued drinking actually lowers blood sugar so the appetite center continues to ask for foods to increase blood sugar levels. You respond by drinking more alcohol and dropping blood sugar levels even lower. Glutamine breaks this cycle by suppressing the sugar-craving messages in the brain and restoring blood sugar to normal levels. The need to drink alcohol to raise blood sugar levels no longer exists and craving wanes.

Much scientific evidence to support the claim that L-glutamine reduces alcohol appetite comes from the late Dr. Roger Williams and colleagues at the University of Texas at Austin. A pioneer in the research of L-glutamine and alcoholism, Dr. Williams, along with associates Drs. Lorene Rogers and Roger Pelton, conducted a number of studies in the 1950's which showed decreased alcohol craving and consumption in animals that were given the amino acid. Drs. Rogers and Pelton then administered L-glutamine to alcoholics who reduced their alcohol intake with the supplement. They also noted the amino acid lowered anxiety levels in the drinkers. More research by Dr. Lorene Rogers involved two groups of alcoholics – one group was given L-glutamine and the other a placebo. She reported the alcoholics given the L-glutamine noticed a reduction in craving, while the alcoholics given the placebo did not. Dr. William Shive, another associate of Dr. Williams, has also studied the effects of L-glutamine on craving. His research concluded it can stop the urge to drink in many but not all alcoholics.

More recently, Dr. Kenneth Blum and associates looked into neurotransmitter deficiencies in alcoholics. They gave several amino acid supplements, including L-glutamine plus a multivitamin with minerals, to some subjects, while others received a placebo. Blum noticed less stress and fewer withdrawal symptoms in the alcoholics taking the amino acid/multivitamin combinations compared to the alcoholics taking the placebo. Less physiological and psychological stress may translate into less drinking desire.

No Daily Value has been established for glutamine. Fish, meat, dairy products, spinach and beans contain the amino acid.

Do not take L-glutamine if you have kidney or liver problems, suffer from Reye's syndrome, if you are pregnant or breastfeeding or if you are healthy and over the age of 55. Best to see your physician prior to taking this amino acid.

L-Tryptophan

Tryptophan is an amino acid important in the production of serotonin, a neurotransmitter which stabilizes mood and regulates sleep. L-tryptophan, the supplemental form of the amino acid, is considered a natural tranquilizer, sleeping aid and an appetite and alcohol craving suppressor.

Drinkers who abuse alcohol tend to suffer from a tryptophan deficiency because alcohol impairs tryptophan from getting to the brain. In the brain, the amino acid is converted to serotonin. Drinkers low on tryptophan are also low on serotonin which is linked to depression and sleeping problems. Negativity, irritability, low self-worth, sleeping disorders, obsessive/compulsive behavior, intolerance to heat and seasonal affective disorder (SAD) are also signs of too little tryptophan.

Adding L-tryptophan to the diet restores serotonin and replaces depression with feelings of well-being. Preliminary research also indicates the amino acid may cut alcohol and food cravings, promote sleep and prevent panic attacks. Stress, migraines, hyperactivity and jet lag are all treated with the supplement.

No Daily Value has been established for tryptophan. Small amounts of the amino acid can be found in meats, brown rice, beans, spinach, peanuts, cottage cheese, pumpkin seeds and soy protein.

Supplements were banned at one time in the United States because of a correlation between a blood disorder and the products containing L-tryptophan. They are now legal and sold over the counter. Too much tryptophan may cause anxiety, headache, sleeping and gastrointestinal disorders. People with asthma should avoid it. It may interact with other medications. Please consult your doctor if you are seriously considering L-tryptophan.

The Craving Game

You started a Craving Diary, now start a Craving Graph. Make a three month graph jotting down Week One, Week Two, Week Three and so on, on the top of the graph. And on the left hand side of the graph record craving intensity with one being the least intense craving and ten being the most intense craving.

At the end of each week average your craving intensity with the information from your Craving Diary and record the average on the Graph. With your craving awareness soaring to new heights, is your desire to drink decreasing or increasing?

Chapter 7
Traditional Herbs to Calm Alcohol Craving

Long before synthetic drugs were developed, Europeans and Native Americans healed with herbs from Mother Nature's pharmacy. Herbal or botanical medicine has been practiced since before recorded history and it refers to the use of flowers, berries, seeds, leaves, bark or roots of a plant to prevent or treat disease. This chapter explores traditional western herbs to cleanse the body, soothe the soul and calm alcohol craving.

Over the last twenty years natural botanical remedies have become increasingly popular and are gaining the acceptance of western medicine. And even though interest in herbal treatments is on the rise, scientific research looking into the efficacy of many plant cures has been neglected. A few herbs, like milk thistle and St. John's wort, are backed by a wealth of evidence proving they work. Most herbs, however, have not been seriously investigated and their active ingredients are not known. Here we must rely on the herbalist's word, based on hundreds of years of observation and use, that preparations given to treat an ailment are effective.

Herbs can be slower acting than processed drugs – many take two to four weeks before you see any difference. And they are often combined with other herbs to increase effectiveness and reduce side effects. Note that the herbs covered here are listed alphabetically in each section, not necessarily in the order of their importance.

Keep in mind there is no government watchdog which regulates the manufacturing or sale of herbs and there is no guarantee as to the safety, purity or potency of an herbal product. Best to consult a qualified herbalist or your herbally-aware physician before considering any remedy – especially if you take any over-the-counter or prescription medication or if you suffer from any pre-existing medical or psychological condition.

First. Cleanse and Nourish Your Body

Dandelion
Taraxacum officinale

Vitamins A, B1, B2, B6, B12, C and D plus zinc, iron, and potassium are just some of the valuable nutrients packed into this purifying plant. Even though most of us consider dandelion just a weed, it has been used for centuries to detoxify and heal the liver and body.

Traditionally, dandelion is given for liver ailments, fever, diarrhea, diabetes, arthritis, gout and eye problems. Native Americans use it to relieve indigestion, heartburn, swelling, kidney and skin conditions.

Today, the herb is used to lower high blood pressure, aid digestion, stimulate appetite and promote urine excretion – all functions vital to ridding yourself of alcohol-related toxins and healing the body. The root is known as an excellent liver cleanser – eliminating impurities from the bloodstream and liver and increasing the flow of bile from the gallbladder to the stomach for good digestion. As a natural diuretic it helps with the excretion of water and salts from the kidneys. The plant is also a rich source of potassium, a mineral which many heavy drinkers are short on. Shouldn't dandelion salad be on your menu tonight?

Even though dandelion is generally considered safe, some people may be allergic to it and it may interact with other medications. If you suffer from gallstones or gall bladder problems, dandelion may not be right for you. Take your interest in this herb to a qualified herbalist or your doctor.

Goldenseal
Hydrastis canadensis

Indigenous to North America, goldenseal has earned the reputation of being a superior blood and liver cleanser. Native Americans used it for skin and eye diseases and introduced it to American settlers.

The herb is a common digestive aid to settle an upset stomach and it is also given to heal a variety of infections, flu, colds, hay fever, pink eye and urinary tract problems. It is thought to improve liver, spleen, pancreas, colon and respiratory functioning. And it is believed to reverse liver damage, produce bile in the gallbladder to help digestion and excrete toxins through sweat and urine. The plant strengthens the immune system overall.

Goldenseal has antibiotic, antiseptic and astringent properties. One of the active ingredients of the plant is berberine which is an all-purpose disinfectant. It kills a wide range of bacteria and parasites, increases your ability to fight infection and enhances the immune system. Other research suggests the herb may also have cardiovascular benefits. It dilates the blood vessels and may help people suffering from irregular heartbeat and heart failure.

Caution – goldenseal should not be taken in large amounts or over a long period of time. Side effects may include nausea, diarrhea and skin, mouth and vaginal irritation with prolonged use. Do not take this remedy if you are pregnant or have high blood pressure. Medical supervision is a must with goldenseal.

Licorice
Glycyrrhiza glaba

Eat candy, purify body? It may not be quite that simple, however we do know licorice has been used not only as a food, but also as a medicine, for thousands of years to prevent and cure illness. People around the world have prescribed licorice or sweet root for everything from colds to stomach problems to skin and liver diseases. Today, it is used for indigestion, ulcers, gastritis, herpes, colic, epilepsy, hepatitis, asthma, chronic fatigue syndrome, menopause and shingles.

Licorice has anti-inflammatory, antiviral and antioxidant characteristics which soothe irritation and stimulate secretions. Glycyrrhizin is one of the active ingredients of the plant thought to provide the healing benefits.

Several Japanese studies indicate the remedy prevents and treats hepatitis. One study, in which patients with hepatitis C were given glycyrrhizin, showed vastly improved liver function after just one month but this improvement diminished as soon as the treatment stopped. Another study looked at people suffering from hepatitis C who received injections of glycyrrhizin with cysteine and glycine over an average of ten years. Results revealed these patients were less prone to cirrhosis and liver cancer than patients on a placebo. The herb is also showing some promise in the treatment of heart disease. Research suggests it reduces blood pressure and "bad" LDL cholesterol.

Too much licorice may be too much of a good thing – leading to fatigue, headache, increased blood pressure, water retention and heart problems. Long term use is not advised. The herb is not recommended for pregnant or breastfeeding women or for people suffering from high blood pressure, diabetes or kidney, liver or heart disease. The plant interacts with many over-the-counter and prescription medications. Seek the advice of a qualified health professional before experimenting with licorice, especially if you suffer from any medical problems or if you take any medication.

Milk Thistle
Silybum marianum

Milk thistle is the herbal superstar when it comes to cleaning, healing and protecting the liver. It has been a liver tonic for ages and is one of the most thoroughly researched medicinal herbs. It blocks harmful toxins from entering the liver, removes impurities from liver cells, rejuvenates injured liver cells and regenerates new ones!

Herbalists prescribe the remedy for alcohol-related liver and spleen problems. Today, it continues to be used to purify and heal the liver damaged by alcohol abuse and has been proven to be an effective treatment for mild to serious liver disease. It also strengthens the immune system of drinkers suffering from chronic alcohol-related liver disease and extends the life span of patients with liver problems.

The active ingredient is silymarin – a powerful antioxidant which prevents free radical damage in the liver. It protects the liver from toxins, including alcohol, and shields the organ from damage caused by fatty liver disease. It improves liver function in people suffering from cirrhosis of the liver and it is a treatment for both hepatitis B and C. Last but not least, silymarin promotes the growth of new liver cells – replacing parts of the liver that have been damaged. The liver is one of the few organs in the body capable of regenerating itself after injury. Research also shows silymarin protects the kidneys and prevents gallstones.

Many studies support milk thistle as an excellent treatment for cirrhosis, chronic hepatitis and alcohol-induced fatty liver. One 1992 study gave high doses of silymarin to 2,637 people with unspecified liver disease over an eight-week period. The patients enjoyed significantly improved liver function by the end of the study. Another 1989 study by Ferenci and colleagues split subjects suffering from cirrhosis of the liver, including subjects suffering from cirrhosis due to alcohol abuse, into two groups. One group received silymarin, while the other group received a placebo. Drinking alcohol was not permitted. The patients treated with the silymarin survived longer than the patients who were given the placebo.

Milk thistle is generally considered safe, but diarrhea may be a side effect. Some medications may interact with this herb. If you suffer from any liver disease, especially hepatitis C, you need to see your physician before taking milk thistle.

Next, Relax and Lift Your Spirits

Passionflower
Passiflora incarnata

Passionflower is native to the Americas and was first used by the Aztecs. Traditionally a calming herb, it is given to relieve anxiety, tension and insomnia. It is also used to treat hypertension, shingles, epilepsy, Parkinson's disease and hyperactive children.

The active ingredient is chrysin. Considered a sedative, it quiets the nervous system and promotes relaxation, mild euphoria and sleep. It may also relax blood vessel spasms – helping to ease the pain of migraines.

In one recent study scientists gave passionflower to thirty-six men and women suffering from generalized anxiety disorder for one month. The subjects found it was just as effective as a popular anti-anxiety prescription drug. Another 1997 study administered an herbal compound containing passionflower with other calming herbs or a placebo to people experiencing anxiety symptoms. The herbal compound with passionflower significantly reduced anxiety symptoms compared to the placebo.

Passionflower is used in many sedatives sold in Europe. Soothing and tranquilizing, Dr. Andrew Weil, founding director of the University of Arizona College of Medicine Center for Integrative Medicine and author of *Natural Health, Natural Medicine*, suggests passionflower as part of a stress reduction program. He considers it much safer than prescription tranquilizers.

Passionflower is generally safe when used correctly but side effects may include nausea, vomiting and rapid heartbeat. Do not take this remedy before driving or operating machinery. Do not take it if you are pregnant or breastfeeding or if you take sedatives or antihistamines. Talk to your herbal professional or doctor if you are passionate about this herb.

St. John's Wort
Hypericum perforatum

Often referred to as "natural Prozac," St. John's wort has been a cure for the blues for over 2,000 years. Herbalists prescribe this antidepressant remedy to elevate and maintain mood. It is recommended for depression and the stress, anxiety and insomnia which may accompany it. There is also some evidence it may curb alcohol craving. Common in Europe and North America, the U.S. National Institutes of Health recognize it as an effective treatment for depression.

Initially, the active ingredients of the plant were thought to be hypericin and hyperforin. Then xanthones and flavonoids were believed to hold the keys to the herb's success. Currently, some researchers think other constituents of the extract are responsible for relieving mild to moderate depression. But even though experts cannot agree on the active ingredient, they do agree the herb increases dopamine production in the brain which promotes feelings of well-being.

In 1996, Linde and associates conducted a meta-analysis of twenty-three randomized trials with 1,757 mildly to moderately depressed patients which was published in the British Medical Journal. Results revealed the extract of the herb proved to be significantly better for mild to moderate depression than a placebo and was just as good as standard antidepressants after an average six week treatment. Linde also noted that only twenty percent of the patients taking St. John's wort suffered side effects compared to over half of those taking prescription antidepressants.

St. John's wort is not only a terrific mood enhancer, it may also have anti-alcohol craving properties too. Researchers at the University of North Carolina School of Medicine at Chapel Hill believe it may prevent alcohol abuse. In 1998, Dr. Amir Rezvani and colleagues conducted several studies with rats, which were selectively bred to prefer alcohol, to see how St. John's wort might affect their drinking behavior. The alcohol-preferring rats were split into two groups – one group was given St. John's wort extract containing hypericin and hyperforin and the other group was not. All of the rats were given free access to water and alcohol for twenty-four hours and their alcohol intake was measured every two hours. Rezvani found the rats receiving the St. John's wort compound drank about fifty percent less alcohol than the animals who did not receive it. The extract significantly reduced alcohol consumption and the animals did not develop a tolerance to the alcohol-curbing effects of the compound.

Rezvani thinks there is a strong biological link between depression and alcoholism and if St. John's wort can alleviate depression, it could also benefit people suffering from alcohol abuse. But he cautions the herb is not a magic bullet because alcoholism is such a complex problem. Still, he thinks a combination of compounds affecting brain chemistry could help individuals motivated to modify their drinking behavior.

St. John's wort is generally considered safe but may cause indigestion, fatigue and restlessness. When taken in high doses it may interfere with the absorption of minerals and cause sun sensitivity. The herb may interact with prescription and over-the-counter medications. The U.S. Food and Drug Administration has issued a public health advisory concerning the interactions of the herb with some medications. It should not be taken with antidepressants. You would be wise to consult your physician if you are serious about St. John's wort.

Skullcap
Scutellaria lateriflora

Native to North America, skullcap is a member of the mint family and has been used as a mild sedative for more than 200 years. Modern herbalists continue to prescribe it to settle nerves and relieve anxiety, tension and insomnia. Headaches, muscle spasms, seizure disorders and anorexia are also treated with skullcap.

Little scientific information is available about this remedy. Animal studies suggest scutellarian, one of the active ingredients of the herb, is responsible for its calming effect. To date, human studies have not been conducted to determine the effectiveness of skullcap as a tranquilizer.

Skullcap is considered safe when properly prescribed, but liver damage has been linked to this plant. This is probably because some skullcap products contain the herb germander which causes liver damage.

Too much skullcap may cause twitching, confusion and irregular heartbeat. Do not take this herb if you are pregnant or breastfeeding. Because of the sedative effects of skullcap, do not take it if you are already taking anti-anxiety, antihistamine or sleep medications. Even though there are no reports of interactions with other medications, exercise caution because of the lack of safety information about this herb. See a qualified herbalist or herbally-aware healthcare professional before you consider skullcap.

Valerian
Valeriana officinale

Valerian is known as "nature's tranquilizer" and translates from Latin as meaning "well-being" – in spite of its awful smell. Europeans have used it to settle the nerves since the sixteenth century and even today it is the most widely used sedative in Europe. Traditional herbalists give it for a variety of nervous disorders, including anxiety, depression, restlessness, insomnia, epilepsy and hysteria. It is also suggested for muscle spasms and menstrual cramps.

Mild and not habit forming, some scientists believe valepotriates are the active ingredients responsible for its tranquilizing effect. Others, however, cannot agree on the active ingredient. But they all do agree on valerian's success in reducing anxiety and stress. In a 1997 study of 182 people suffering from anxiety, some were given a valerian root compound while others were given a placebo. The valerian group enjoyed significant relief from anxiety symptoms compared to the subjects taking the placebo.

Studies have also shown valerian not only improves sleep quality, but it causes one to fall asleep faster too. A 1982 study with 128 patients, who considered themselves poor sleepers, concluded the extract of the herb caused the subjects to fall asleep faster and enhanced the quality of their sleep. A 1988 Swedish study administered valerian root to one group of people and a placebo to another group. Eighty-nine percent of the valerian subjects reported a vast improvement in sleep and forty-four percent reported "perfect sleep" compared to the placebo group.

Dr. Andrew Weil thinks valerian is one of the safest sedatives around and may be helpful for people interested in eliminating addictive behaviors. He believes it is more effective than other herbal sedatives, like hops and skullcap, and should be in every family's medicine cabinet.

Valerian is generally considered safe, but side effects may include stomach upset and overstimulation. Do not take this herb before driving or operating machinery. Long-term use is not recommended and do not take this remedy if you are taking any prescription tranquilizers or antidepressants. See a qualified herbalist or your doctor before testing valerian.

Now, Calm the Craving

Evening Primrose Oil
Oenothera biennis

Evening primrose oil is a cureall for a number of health problems and is sometimes prescribed for alcoholism and alcohol craving. Native to North America, it alleviates the depression associated with problem drinking and protects the liver and kidneys from damage caused by chronic alcohol abuse.

Traditionally, the oil is prescribed for stomach and respiratory ailments. It is also given for arthritis, allergies, acne, eczema, diabetes, obesity, PMS, menopause, osteoporosis, high blood pressure, heart disease, multiple sclerosis, neuropathy, schizophrenia and hyperactivity.

The seed oil is a good source of gamma linoleic acid (GLA) which plays an important role in brain functioning. GLA is an essential fatty acid which promotes the production of prostaglandins. Prostaglandins regulate blood pressure and have a profound effect on the nervous system and behavior.

Chronic heavy drinking cuts GLA and prostaglandin production which may cause depression and trigger alcohol craving and abuse. Evening primrose oil, rich in GLA and a precursor to prostaglandins, may relieve that depression and the need to drink. Some animal studies confirm the oil reduces alcohol appetite. More research with humans is needed.

Evening primrose oil is considered safe if used correctly. Rare side effects may include nausea and headache. Do not take this remedy if you have any seizure disorder – it may induce seizures. Do not take this remedy if you are pregnant or breastfeeding – it may induce early labor and be harmful to the baby. The oil interacts with a number of prescription drugs. To be on the safe side, consult your herbalist or physician before trying evening primrose oil.

Kava Kava
Piper methysticum

Kava kava grows in the South Pacific Islands where it is considered sacred. The plant is related to the pepper family and its Latin name translates as "intoxicating pepper." The herb calms anxiety and lifts mood without impairing thought processes and preliminary research suggests it may also curb alcohol craving.

Herbalists give kava to step on anxiety and depression and to promote relaxation, euphoria and restful sleep. It is also used for tension headaches, to soothe sore muscles and muscle spasms and to prevent seizures.

Kavapyrones are thought to be the active ingredient of the plant. Also known as kavalactones, the substance works on the central nervous system, relaxes the skeletal muscles and helps regulate and normalize high heart rate, blood pressure and body temperature associated with anxiety. The result is decreased anxiety and depression and increased relaxation and better sleep.

Individuals who have taken kava enjoy a gradual lessening of anxiety symptoms without any side effects. A 1991 study by Kinzler and colleagues gave one group of patients suffering from anxiety kava extract and another group a placebo. The four week study showed the subjects taking the kava extract enjoyed a significant improvement and reduction in anxiety symptoms compared to those taking the placebo. Nervousness, headache, dizziness and palpitations associated with anxiety were reduced and no side effects were reported. In 2000, Pittler and Ernst at the University of Exeter Department of Complementary Medicine in England, also concluded that kava extract was superior in treating anxiety compared to placebos. Other research suggests kava may be just as useful for treating anxiety as pharmaceutical anti-anxiety and antidepressant medications. Dr. Andrew Weil feels kava is a natural alternative to synthetic antidepressants which may be addictive.

Preliminary findings confirm kava may also reduce alcohol craving. Scientists think kavapyrones bind to areas in the brain associated with craving and addiction. Two studies reported in 2001 showed subjects given kava felt a reduced craving for their drug of choice and drinkers taking kava abstained for longer periods than drinkers not taking kava. More work is needed.

The U.S. Food and Drug Administration has issued a warning about kava causing liver damage. Germany and Canada have taken kava off the market for this reason. High doses may cause upset stomach, intoxication, sleepiness or liver damage. Do not take kava before driving or operating machinery or if you are pregnant or breastfeeding. Do not take kava if you suffer from serious liver or alcohol problems or if you take any other medications. Check with your doctor before deciding if this herb is right for you.

The Craving Game

You've been keeping track of your craving and the intensity of your craving. Now start keeping track of how your desire to drink affects your alcohol consumption. From now on, record the number of drinks you have for each drinking occasion. Is there a correlation between your drinking desire and your alcohol intake?

Chapter 8
Homeopathic Remedies Set You Free From the Need to Drink

Stimulating the natural healing ability of the body to prevent or cure illness is the goal of homeopathic medicine. Developed in Europe by German physician Samuel Hahnemann in the nineteenth century, it teaches every person possesses a vital energy force and a balance of this force leads to good health and mental, emotional and physical freedom. Disease develops when this energy is not in balance and limits this freedom. Invigorating your self-healing responses with homeopathic remedies to cleanse the body, brighten the mood and free you from the need to drink is the goal of this chapter.

Homeopathy is based on three principles. First, the belief that "like cures like" – meaning a remedy which produces symptoms of a disease will cure that disease if taken in small doses. Second, the more diluted a homeopathic medicine is, the greater curative power and fewer side effects it will have. Third, each patient is a unique individual and presents a unique set of symptoms requiring a unique combination of remedies to address mental, emotional and physical factors which will encourage the healing process.

The traditional homeopath does not treat alcohol abuse specifically. They treat the individual suffering from it and believe improving the drinker's physiological and psychological condition with homeopathic medicine is one way to become less dependent on alcohol.

Then, when the drinker's needs are met and they feel better, they will no longer need alcohol and engage in destructive drinking.

When treating a chronic disease determining a patient's personality or "constitution" is a must in homeopathy. Physical, emotional and mental factors make up a person's constitution and a patient classified as a certain constitutional type benefits the most from taking remedies associated with that type. But knowing your constitution is not required when treating acute illnesses, like a cold or the flu, or symptoms of an illness, like a fever or cough. Since the purpose of this book is to relieve common symptoms and causes of alcohol craving and abuse, determining your constitution would be helpful but is not essential to benefit from a homeopathic approach.

Over 1,300 substances derived from animal, vegetable and mineral sources make up the homeopathic pharmacy. These medicines do not create a chemical reaction in the body, like drugs, but stimulate the system to better cope with stress and illness. Some preparations originate from dangerous substances like strychnine, snake venom and arsenic. But when prepared as a homeopathic remedy they are highly diluted and non-toxic. And even though modern clinical research has shown homeopathic medicines are significantly more effective than a placebo, little has been written about homeopathic cures for alcohol craving specifically.

Keep in mind certain rules are followed when administering homeopathic remedies. Remember – the remedy that produces the same symptoms as the disease is selected. Only one medicine is given at a time. If there is improvement, wait and allow the preparation to work. As long as there is improvement there is no need to continue taking the remedy. If improvement slows or stops, take another dose. If no response is seen, try another medicine.

Official homeopathic remedies are considered drugs under federal law and must meet guidelines developed by the U.S. Food and Drug

Administration and the American Homeopathic Pharmacists Association. A substance must have "provings" (case studies) it produces the symptoms of a disease for which it is prescribed and it must meet manufacturing specifications set by the Homoeopathic Pharmacopoeia of the United States (HPUS). This organization offers information on manufacturing procedures, dosage, administration and labeling. Look for HPUS initials on the medicine label insuring legal standards for purity, quality and strength have been met.

If you choose to experiment with homeopathic remedies, you may be taking your life in your hands. The wrong prescription or dose could make you very sick or even kill you. Take your interest in homeopathic medicine to a licensed homeopath or your physician to derive the greatest benefits from it.

First, Concentrate on Physical Health

Aconitum Napellus

Aconitum should be included in everyone's first aid kit because of its ability to minimize shock, fever and infection. This plant remedy, also known as monkshood, is widely used to treat physical and emotional stress. In addition to relieving the physical discomfort a drinker may suffer when cutting back on alcohol, aconitum may also soothe the restlessness and irritability associated with drinking less. Aconitum types are fearful and anxious and may suffer from heart palpitations.

Homeopathic healers give aconitum for fevers, colds, coughs, headaches, aches and pains, ear, eye and throat problems. It is also used for anxiety, fear, palpitations, panic attacks and insomnia. What better remedy than aconitum when coming down from too much alcohol?

Alkaloids found in the perennial have anti-inflammatory and pain-killing properties and the active ingredient is aconitine. The root of the plant is highly toxic – just one teaspoon can paralyze the heart muscle – but when prepared as a homeopathic medicine it is not considered dangerous.

Professional advice from a homeopath or doctor is a must for correct prescription and dosage of this remedy.

Arnica Montana

Native Americans and Europeans have used a plant known as leopard's bane for muscle pain centuries before it was refined as a homeopathic preparation. It is also considered an excellent first aid remedy because it reduces the pain, shock, bleeding and bruising following injuries. Arnica types like to be left alone. They do not like to be touched and feel better with movement.

Traditionally, arnica is prescribed for physiological and psychological shock. Fever, muscle pain, headaches, boils, osteoarthritis, whooping cough and physical and mental trauma are all cared for with this medicine. It is also given to relieve grief and remorse.

Arnica has anti-inflammatory qualities, improves circulation, controls bleeding, suppresses swelling, speeds healing and resists infection. Modern uses of the remedy include treating pain, headaches, abscesses and angina.

Even though the homeopathic substance is highly diluted and considered safe when used according to directions, the unprocessed plant is poisonous even in small doses. Talk to your homeopathic practitioner or physician before you consider this remedy.

Arsenicum Album

Feeling restless, anxious, exhausted? Tummy upset? Arsenicum album, a mineral remedy, may be just what the homeopath orders. Arsenicum calms the nervous and digestive systems – making it the perfect medicine to get back on the wellness track. Arsenicum types are ambitious perfectionists always worried about their health. They are neat and meticulous and suffer from anxiety and restlessness. They prefer warm, fatty foods, coffee and alcohol.

Homeopaths recommend arsenicum for gastrointestinal and emotional problems. Indigestion, diarrhea, vomiting, headaches, colds, hay fever, stomach flu and gastroenteritis are all treated with the mineral. It is also given for exhaustion, restlessness, anxiety, fear, worry and alcoholism.

Arsenicum album is derived from arsenic oxide – yes, as in arsenic poison. But it can be beneficial when prepared as a homeopathic remedy and given in small, diluted doses. Avoid arsenicum album if you are pregnant or breastfeeding. Consult a licensed homeopath or your healthcare professional for correct prescription and dosage, especially if you are taking any other medications or suffer from allergies.

Bryonia Alba

A hangover remedy, bryonia was popular with the ancient Greeks and Romans. Also known as wild hops, Augustus Caesar wore a wreath made from the plant because he thought it protected him from lightning during thunderstorms. Bryonia types suffer from fatigue and irritability. They feel exhausted and do not like to speak or move when sick.

Bryonia is prescribed for fevers, nausea, flu, colds, coughs, osteoarthritis and pneumonia. It is also given to relieve the upset stomach, pounding headache, irritability and aches and pains of a hangover. Relief is on the way with bryonia!

The unrefined plant can be poisonous and overdosing may cause vomiting, convulsions and kidney and liver damage. However, the homeopathic medicine contains an extremely small amount of the herb and it is highly diluted. Professional supervision by a homeopathic healer or your physician is required before trying this remedy.

Chamomilla

Wild chamomile, which is the source of this homeopathic remedy, has been used for ages to relax the nervous system and aid digestion. Chamomilla constitutional types are supersensitive and become irritable when uncomfortable. Symptoms worsen at night and with heat.

Homeopathy suggests chamomilla for all kinds of stomach and digestive ailments and as a sedative for emotional upset. Diarrhea, constipation, nausea, fevers, migraines, arthritis, bronchitis, asthma, cough, colic, teething and menstrual problems are all cared for with the remedy. It is also given to alleviate stress, soothe anger and irritability and to promote sleep.

Wild chamomile is an antiseptic bacteria fighter and a natural pain reliever. Today, it is used to treat a variety of conditions, including headaches, colds, acne, burns, hay fever, sinusitis, peptic ulcers, gastroenteritis and skin diseases. It dulls the pain of childbirth and is a common stress, headache and digestion medicine in Europe.

Animal studies show chamomile reduces inflammation and muscle spasms and initiates healing. People suffering from liver disease and AIDS may benefit from the remedy. It is one of the few substances capable of regenerating new liver cells. In one study, active ingredients azulene and guaiazulene helped form new liver tissue in rats who had part of the liver removed.

Chamomilla is considered safe but allergic reactions are common. Side effects may include stomachache, itching, hives, shortness of breath and anaphylactic shock – a condition which can be fatal and requires immediate medical attention. Do not take this medicine if you are taking sedatives or blood-thinning medication. Best to see your homeopath or doctor before getting serious about chamomilla.

Lycopodium

About 360 million years ago giant club moss forests covered the earth. This ancient club moss then evolved into a small evergreen, lycopodium, which has been a cureall since the Middle Ages. Throughout history it has been offered to treat a number of ailments – from digestive, liver and kidney diseases to worry and indecision. Lycopodium types may seem self-confident but are actually insecure. They also tend to be irritable, overbearing and easily intimidated by people they think are powerful.

Homeopathic practitioners give lycopodium to relieve indigestion, nausea, vomiting and constipation. It flushes impurities from the blood, liver and kidneys and it is also recommended for headaches, flu, sore throat and chronic fatigue syndrome. This preparation soothes a negative mood and it is often prescribed for anxiety, irritability, apprehension and insomnia – feelings which may have started you drinking in the first place and feelings you may experience when trying to cut down.

The plant has diuretic and sedative properties and modern uses of the medicine include the treatment of digestive, urinary tract and skin problems. Lycopodium is generally considered safe with no side effects reported.

Next, Concentrate on Mental Health

Avena Sativa

Not feeling your oats? The calming antidepressant features of this wild oat remedy will settle you down and help you achieve a comfortable emotional balance – even if you are reducing your alcohol consumption. Oats have been given to heal the nervous system for thousands of years and offer a myriad of health benefits – making avena sativa a favorite among homeopaths.

The oat preparation is prescribed to alleviate depression, anxiety, nervous exhaustion, insomnia and impotence. It strengthens the nervous system and produces feelings of relaxation and well-being. It is considered an excellent cure for hangovers, headaches and restlessness caused by overdrinking. Avena is also believed to improve concentration, stamina and endurance and promote good health in general.

The remedy is crammed full of nutrients – vitamins, protein, calcium, iron, potassium, magnesium and fat. Oat fiber builds strong bones and teeth and is an important digestive aid – soothing gastrointestinal conditions. It also lowers blood pressure, cholesterol and blood sugar levels and prevents heart disease and cancer. With all of these pluses, isn't it time you get excited about that bowl of oatmeal in the morning?

Avena is considered quite safe but people who are gluten sensitive should not take it.

Calcarea Carbonica

Processed from the mother of pearl layer of oyster shell, this mineral medicine is a treatment for a variety of different health problems. It is thought to soothe the spirit and promote healing and some think it may even reduce alcohol craving. Calcarea types are quiet, hard-working individuals who are restless, irritable and afraid of the dark. They are practical and sensitive and want security.

Homeopathy prescribes the remedy for mental and physical exhaustion and it is given to relieve anxiety, fear, insomnia and obsessive-compulsive behavior. Calcarea lends nutritional support to the skin, bones and glands and it is often recommended for colds, coughs, digestive ailments, diarrhea, constipation and arthritis. Chills, night sweats, teething, pituitary and thyroid problems are also treated with the preparation.

Calcarea is considered safe with no side effects when properly prescribed.

Ignatia

This remedy is derived from the seeds of the St. Ignatius bean plant which contains strychnine poison. It is thought to restore psychological balance and it is commonly used to treat emotional disorders. Ignatia types are sensitive and high-strung. They suffer from rapid mood changes and feelings of loss and disappointment.

Traditionally, ignatia is given to calm negative states, including depression, anger, fear, worry, grief and insomnia. It is also used for fevers, headaches, cough, throat and menstrual ailments.

Be careful if you consider ignatia. The unprocessed plant is poisonous and a small dose may result in convulsions and death. The homeopathic preparation, however, contains a very small amount of the substance and is not considered dangerous. Visit your homeopath or doctor if you are interested in ignatia.

Pulsatilla

Pulsatilla is an anti-anxiety, antidepressant remedy which slows breathing, reduces arterial tension and dilates the pupils. Originating from the windflower plant, it is a multipurpose medicine used to treat many health conditions. Pulsatilla types are shy, insecure, emotional individuals. They are homebodies who need lots of support and comforting. They cry easily and feel lonely and isolated in the outside world.

Homeopathic healers offer pulsatilla for depression, anxiety and digestive, sinus, ear and eye problems. It is also given for colds, flu, acne, migraines and rheumatism. Pulsatilla is recommended for women suffering from menstrual problems and it is considered a woman's remedy. In France it is taken for insomnia.

Exercise caution with pulsatilla. While there are no known side effects when administered in small homeopathic doses, the unrefined perennial is toxic and can be fatal when taken in large doses. Pregnant and breastfeeding women should avoid the preparation. Seek the advice of a qualified homeopath or your physician before you get serious about pulsatilla.

Staphysagria

Another popular homeopathic remedy, staphysagria is made from the stavesacre plant which many consider nature's pain reliever. It is believed this medicine reduces the pain from illness caused by suppressed emotions, especially anger and grief, and it helps to maintain an emotional balance without repressing one's feelings. Staphysagria types are thin-skinned, conscientious individuals. They tend to avoid confrontations and are especially sensitive to injustice and betrayal.

Homeopathy prescribes staphysagria for emotional and physical trauma resulting from injury, surgery or childbirth. Nervous problems, depression, irritability, headaches, sciatica, neuritis, eye and urinary tract disorders are also treated with the remedy. It is commonly given for alcohol withdrawal symptoms.

Staphysagria is generally considered safe with no reported side effects when used correctly.

Now, Crush the Craving

Lachesis

An animal substance derived from Bushmaster snake venom, lachesis is considered an "intense" remedy used to treat a number of ailments, including alcohol craving. It is believed this medicine restores equilibrium and promotes well-being. Lachesis types are smart and creative. They are very verbal and may be manipulative. Jealousy and revenge are also personality characteristics.

Some homeopaths look to lachesis to reduce the desire to drink alcohol. It is also used to treat depression, irritability, headaches, angina, delirium tremens and nervous system disorders. Lachesis thins the blood and it is recommended for vascular and circulatory problems. It is often given for women's complaints – PMS, hot flashes and menopause.

The homeopathic preparation is considered safe when properly prescribed. High doses, however, may be harmful even life threatening. Consult your homeopath or doctor before fooling with lachesis.

Nux Vomica

Nux vomica should be your remedy of choice if physical and mental stress are triggering your alcohol craving and problem drinking. This medicine is made from the strychnine tree – yes, as in the deadly poison – but when taken in small doses, it may take the edge off of drinking desire.

Nux types are sensitive, ambitious, hardworking, impatient people. They feel frustrated and angry when things don't go their way which may lead to too much drinking and illness. Nux types may not only drink too much alcohol, they may eat too much food, drink too much coffee, smoke too many cigarettes and do other drugs. They are prone to indigestion and hypertension. Nux is most often prescribed for men.

Homeopaths calm anger, stress, irritability and oversensitivity and restore psychological balance with nux vomica. It is also given for hangovers, headaches, digestive problems, insomnia and back and joint pain which may be brought on by overindulgence. It helps in many different ways so you no longer need alcohol.

Nux is one of the few homeopathic remedies to be studied as a treatment for alcohol abuse. N.C. Sukul and colleagues at Visva-Bharati University in India conducted animal studies and discovered the preparation reduces voluntary alcohol consumption in rats. More research with human subjects is needed to explore its anti-alcohol effect.

Nux vomica is generally considered safe. Even though the homeopathic substance is non-toxic, it is made from strychnine poison which produces muscle spasms and can result in death. You would be wise to seek the advice of a qualified homeopathic healer or physician before experimenting with nux.

Quercus Glandius Spiritus

This very old, forgotten remedy was used to curb alcohol craving in the early days of homeopathy. Also known as Antidote Q, by the common name English oak and by the botanical name Quercus robur, it was not only given to step on drinking desire, but to treat gout, liver and spleen diseases as well. This homeopathic preparation is a tincture made from acorns and alcohol.

Case studies presented by James Crompton Burnett, a nineteenth century homeopath and author of over twenty books on homeopathic medicine, suggest quercus does indeed reduce alcohol craving. One man suffering from alcoholism, gout and bronchitis with an enlarged liver and spleen took the tincture three times a day and claimed it took away his desire for alcohol. Another man, also an alcohol abuser with an enlarged liver and spleen, depressed and nervous, started quercus. After six weeks Burnett pronounced him "well." Burnett offered three more case studies of individuals suffering from alcohol abuse and alcohol-related health problems who were given quercus. Each patient recovered after taking the remedy. Burnett did not maintain quercus cures alcoholism, but he did consider it to be an "antidote to the alcoholic state" and helpful in reducing alcohol appetite.

William Boericke, author of *Homeopathic Materia Medica* and *A Thousand Remedies*, also claimed quercus "takes away craving for alcohol" and removes "the effects of alcohol." He stated the tincture is a treatment for "gout alcoholism, pain in pit of stomach, tottering gaits, hands quiver, craving of wine."

No information on the safety of quercus is available. A homeopath or physician's supervision is required before testing this little-known remedy.

The Craving Game

What's your homeopathic constitutional type? Go to the library, dig into homeopathy and find out. Then determine what remedies are best suited to your personality so you can eliminate the need to drink.

Part Four:
EASTERN APPROACHES
TO BEAT ALCOHOL CRAVING

Chapter 9

Ancient Chinese Secrets to Quiet Drinking Desire

Over 7,000 herbs have been documented by the Chinese to have positive health benefits! Chinese herbal medicine is centuries old and an important branch of traditional Chinese medicine. Written records of Chinese herbal medicine date back to about 3500 BC and the first book on herbs, the *Agriculture Emperors Materia Medica*, was written in China about 200 BC. Chinese herbs to detoxify the body, soothe the spirit and quiet drinking desire are unearthed in this chapter.

Traditional Chinese medicine is based on the concept of qi (chi), a vital energy or life force which flows through the body. Qi is made up of "yin-yang" – yin is negative energy and yang is positive energy – and it circulates throughout the body via twelve meridians which correspond to different organs. When qi is in balance, good health and resistance to stress and illness result. When qi is not in balance, one is susceptible to disease. The goal of Chinese medicine is to equalize qi and herbal medicine is one of many ways to do that.

The Chinese believe the liver houses the soul and the heart houses the spirit. Alcohol craving and abuse are thought to be caused by a qi deficiency in the liver creating fire and heat. And depression, anxiety, irritability and insomnia – states which may drive one to drink – are linked to a qi deficiency in both the liver and the heart. Herbs that restore and invigorate qi in the liver and heart meridians and clear the fire and heat

109

associated with alcohol abuse are commonly prescribed to treat drinking desire and problem drinking.

Chinese herbs and herbal formulas are made from vegetable, animal and mineral sources and come in many different forms: teas, powders, ointments, liquors, porridges, poultices and pillows. Each herb is classified according to four different properties: energy, flavor, movement and the particular meridian in the body it affects. There are five herb flavors. Pungent herbs encourage blood and qi circulation and are given for superficial problems. Sweet herbs are used to treat deficiencies, toxicity, pain and acute illnesses, like a cold or the flu. Sour herbs stop the loss of bodily fluids and are recommended for perspiration and diarrhea. Salty herbs soften and lubricate and are used for constipation and swellings. And bitter herbs act as laxatives and are offered to reduce fever and clear heat.

Some Chinese herbs have scientific evidence to support their effectiveness and some do not. And many herbs are not used alone, but in combination with other herbs to make up a formula. Exercise caution if you experiment with any herb. Side effects and interactions with other herbs and medications may be hazardous to your health. Best to take your interest in Chinese herbs to a qualified Chinese herbalist or a western medicine physician with expertise in this area.

First, Clear Heat and Detoxify

Bai Shao
Paeonia lactiflora

This sour, bitter, cool herb clears heat and toxins from the blood and liver and revitalizes liver qi. Commonly known as white peony root, it affects the liver and spleen meridians.

Traditional Chinese herbalists give this remedy to soothe the liver, relieve pain and treat sores and infections. Believed to restore blood and liver functions, it is also used for headaches, sore throat, urinary tract infections, gallbladder problems, jaundice and cancer. Considered a woman's herb because it helps regulate menstruation and the female hormonal cycle, men also use it as a blood cleanser. Many think it promotes beautiful skin and long life.

Bai shao has antibacterial, anti-inflammatory, antiviral, pain-relieving and tranquilizing properties. The herb stimulates circulation and strengthens the immune system. Today, it is also used to treat leukemia, appendicitis and snake bites.

Side effects may include skin rash and difficulty breathing. You should not use this remedy if you are pregnant or breastfeeding. Consult a qualified Chinese healer or your doctor before considering bai shao.

Chai Hu
Bupleurum chinense

Bitter, pungent and cool, chai hu is one of the most popular liver rejuvenators in China. Also known as hare's ear or bupleurum, it is often combined with other herbs to create a formula helpful for liver problems. It affects the liver and gallbladder meridians.

Chai hu is prescribed to clear heat, sedate the liver and invigorate liver qi. It is considered one of the best herbs to treat liver diseases, including cirrhosis and hepatitis. Lifting depression is another common use of the remedy. It is also given for fevers, infections, indigestion, irregular menstruation and pain and bloat in the chest and abdomen.

Chai hu has antiviral, antibacterial, anti-inflammatory and pain-killing qualities. Saikosaponins are the active ingredients of the herb and test tube studies found they prevent the growth of liver cancer cells. Human trials have shown a Japanese medicine formula known as sho-saiko-to, with chai hu being the main ingredient, helps reduce the symptoms and liver enzyme levels in people suffering from chronic viral hepatitis. The formula has also been shown to decrease the risk of developing liver cancer in people with chronic viral hepatitis. And sho-saiko-to is also credited with relieving the symptoms and severity of cirrhosis of the liver and preventing liver cancer in patients suffering from cirrhosis. Test tube studies have shown this Japanese formula, in addition to inhibiting the growth of liver cancer cells, also inhibits the growth of the HIV virus and increases the effectiveness of some anti-HIV virus medications. Keep in mind these results cannot be attributed to chai hu alone because this medicine also contains other herbs.

Side effects of this remedy may include headache, dizziness, nausea and vomiting when taken in large doses. It is not recommended for pregnant or breastfeeding women. To be on the safe side, take your interest in chai hu to a qualified Chinese herbalist or your physician.

Gou Teng
Uncaria rhyncophylla

Sweet and cold, gou teng clears heat and calms the liver making it a widely used remedy for liver ailments and depression. Commonly known as cat's claw, it affects the liver and heart meridians.

Besides treating liver and mood problems, gou teng is prescribed by Chinese practitioners for headaches, dizziness, convulsions, spasms and tremors. It is also given to reduce high blood pressure.

The herb has antiviral, anti-inflammatory and sedative properties. The active ingredients are alkaloids and nicotinic acid which lower the heart rate and have a diuretic effect. Gou teng is thought to stimulate the immune system.

Side effects of this remedy may include bleeding and symptoms of low blood pressure. Anyone suffering from tuberculosis or a blood clotting disorder should avoid gou teng. Anyone who has an autoimmune disease should avoid it. Do not take this herb if you are pregnant or breastfeeding. Gou teng may interact with other medications. Consult a qualified Chinese medicine professional or an herbally-aware doctor before testing this herb.

Jin Yin Hua
Lonicera japonica

Clearing heat, eliminating toxins and promoting vitality and long life makes jin yin hua a favorite body/soul herb in Chinese medicine. Also known as honeysuckle, this sweet, cool herb affects the heart, lung, spleen and stomach meridians.

Traditionally used to cleanse and nourish the blood and clear internal heat, herbalists prescribe it for fevers, infections, abscesses, allergies, sore throat, hemorrhoids and obesity.

Containing potassium, magnesium and calcium, the flower has antibacterial, anti-inflammatory and diuretic characteristics. It is believed to protect the liver and lower blood pressure and cholesterol levels. Today, jin yin yua is also used to treat hepatitis, respiratory infections and rheumatoid arthritis.

Long term use of this remedy is not recommended. Check with your herbalist or healthcare provider before experimenting with jin yin hua.

Pu Gong Ying
Taraxacum mongolicum

Dandelion again! Western herbalists are not the only ones to take advantage of this purifying plant to detoxify and treat liver disease. This sweet, bitter, cold herb affects the liver and stomach meridians.

Chinese herbal medicine recommends it to clear heat from the liver, cleanse the blood and remove toxins from the body. Liver, kidney and gallbladder ailments, indigestion, constipation, bruises, gout, diabetes and cancer are all treated with pu gong ying. Chinese healers use the whole dandelion plant versus western herbalists who use only the root.

This potent detoxifying and decongestive remedy is rich in minerals and vitamins A, B and C. It stimulates bile and urine output which rids the body of impurities, including dangerous by-products associated with alcohol, drugs and junk food.

Pu gong ying is considered safe, but some people may be allergic to it. Medical supervision is required before taking this herb.

Wu Wei Dze
Schizandra chinensis

Wu wei dze means "five taste fruit" in Chinese because it is the only herb considered to have all five basic flavors: sweet, sour, bitter, pungent and salty, even though sour is the predominant taste. This sour, warm herb is thought to balance energy and rejuvenate the body and soul. Also known as magnolia vine, it affects the heart, kidney, liver and lung meridians.

Wu wei dze is traditionally given to purify the body and calm the spirit. It is believed to eliminate toxins from the liver, reduce sweating while generating bodily fluids and strengthen the lungs and kidneys. It is prescribed for infections, headaches, asthma, coughs, diarrhea and irritable bowel syndrome. The herb is also thought to relieve stress, irritability, palpitations and insomnia. It is considered an aphrodisiac and is an ingredient in many longevity formulas.

Wu wei dze has antioxidant and antibacterial properties. The active ingredients are lignans and oils in the fruit of the plant. The lignans are powerful antioxidants – scavenging free radicals which cause disease and aging. It appears lignans may also guard the liver by promoting glutathione production in liver cells. Glutathione is also a strong antioxidant. Plus, wu wei dze is an adaptogen – a substance which normalizes organ functions and supports physiological and psychological health. Adaptogens shield you from physical and mental stress and strengthen the immune system.

The herb has special liver-healing qualities. Pharmacological studies have shown it protects and improves the overall functioning of the liver. And research in China found it effectively treated chemical and viral hepatitis. In one study, wu wei dze powder was given to 102 patients suffering from hepatitis. Over seventy percent of the patients enjoyed a return to normal liver enzyme levels with no problems over an average twenty-five day treatment. Other research also suggests the remedy may reduce fatigue, increase strength and enhance work performance and the immune system.

Side effects may include indigestion, skin rash and restlessness. Take your interest in wu wei dze to a qualified Chinese practitioner or your physician.

Next, Calm the Spirit

He Huan Pi
Albizia julibrissin

An antidepressant, he huan pi soothes emotions and enhances mood. Also known as albizzia flower or mimosa tree bark, the Chinese believe it nourishes the heart and the body. This sweet, neutral herb affects the heart and liver meridians.

Chinese herbalists prescribe this remedy to quiet the mind and relieve depression, anxiety and stress. It is given for any emotional upset, including extreme anger, great loss or a broken heart. He huan pi is also used to treat fear, worry, paranoia and sleeplessness. The herb is thought to dull pain, promote circulation and lift the spirits. Modern uses of he huan pi include the treatment of insomnia and bacterial liver infections.

Generally, this remedy is considered safe with no precautions or side effects reported. Consult a Chinese medicine professional or your doctor before proceeding with he huan pi.

Hu Po
Pinites succinifer

Translated from Chinese as "tiger's soul", all of Asia believes sweet, neutral hu po has healing and supernatural powers. Also known as the mineral amber, it sedates the kidneys and reduces heat in the bladder. It affects the bladder, heart and liver meridians.

Hu po is considered a mild and safe tranquilizer which reduces stress, tension, anxiety, irritability and insomnia. It is also given for palpitations, convulsions, epilepsy and abdominal pain. Chinese practitioners think it invigorates the blood, cuts swelling, encourages healing and improves memory, alertness and concentration.

Amber is fossilized tree sap and it comes in many different grades. The best amber for medicinal purposes is reddish or dark brown. Today, it is still thought to be an excellent sedative – especially good for getting to sleep.

Hu po is considered safe with no precautions or side effects reported. Always best to seek the advice of a qualified Chinese herbalist or your physician before trying any herb.

Long Gu
Stegodon orientalis

Long gu is a mineral remedy processed from the fossilized bones of prehistoric deer, oxen, rhinoceros and mastodon. This sweet, neutral preparation, also known as dragon's bone, calms the liver and the heart producing relaxation and tranquility. Long gu affects the liver, heart, kidney and large intestine meridians.

Traditionally, it is given to settle excitability and to stabilize the spirit. Anxiety, tension, anger, frustration, emotional upset, palpitations and insomnia are all treated with the mineral. In addition to its use as a sedative, it is often prescribed for diarrhea, frequent urination and excessive perspiration.

Long gu is rich in calcium and other minerals – soothing the nerves and muscles. Today, it continues to be a widely used tranquilizer and is said to benefit anyone suffering from the ups and downs of modern day living.

This remedy is never used alone but in combination with other herbs, depending on the problem at hand. It is considered very safe and no side effects have been reported. Consult your Chinese healer for more information about long gu.

Mu Li
Concha ostreae

Oyster shell again! Homeopathy and Chinese herbal medicine have this mineral in common when treating mood and emotional problems. This salty, cool remedy is given to quiet the spirit and it affects the liver and kidney meridians.

Mu li is used to sedate the liver – reducing yang energy and nourishing yin energy. It is prescribed for anxiety, restlessness, fear, palpitations and insomnia. Indigestion, headache, fever and tinnitus are also cared for with this mineral.

Oyster shells are cleaned, dried and ground into a powder to produce the remedy. Today, western medicine turns to oyster shell to prevent and treat osteoporosis, colorectal cancer, hypoglycemia, diarrhea and PMS.

Mu li is considered quite safe with no reported side effects.

Yuan Zhi
Polygala tenuifolia

Without a doubt, yuan zhi is one of the most popular depression-fighting remedies in China. Loosely translated, it means "will power and ambition strengthener." Also known as senega root, this bitter, pungent, warm herb affects the heart and lung meridians.

Chinese herbalists believe yuan zhi nurtures the heart and clears and nourishes the lungs. It is recommended to calm the mind and the spirit – relieving anxiety, irritability, stress, palpitations and insomnia. This herb is the main ingredient in many formulas to treat depression. It is also given for respiratory problems, including asthma, bronchitis and whooping cough. Externally, it is used to treat sores, abscesses and painful breasts.

Modern research indicates yuan zhi has antibacterial and tranquilizing properties. It thins the blood and lowers blood pressure. Today, the remedy continues to be used as an expectorant to clear phlegm from the lungs and to heal lung infections.

If you suffer from gastritis, stomach or digestive problems, you should exercise caution with this herb. Consult a qualified Chinese medicine professional or your doctor before experimenting with yuan zhi.

Now, Quiet the Desire to Drink

Dan Shen
Salvia miltiorrhiza

Dan shen is a multipurpose remedy which may curb alcohol craving. Also known as Chinese sage, red sage and "red ginseng" – not because it's a member of the ginseng family, but because of the red color of its roots – this cool, bitter herb affects the liver and heart meridians.

Traditional Chinese medicine gives it to clear heat, cool and nourish the blood and to soothe the spirit. It is frequently prescribed for irritability, restlessness, palpitations and sleeping problems. The herb is thought to stimulate circulation and build the immune system and it is also used for fevers, heart disease, menstrual and skin conditions.

Modern research suggests it decreases the desire to drink and alcohol consumption. Other studies support it as a treatment for liver diseases, including cirrhosis and chronic hepatitis B. There is also some evidence it may be helpful for heart problems, chest pain, chronic bronchitis and Alzheimer's disease.

Scientists at the University of Cagliari in Italy have conducted a number of animal studies showing dan shen reduces alcohol craving and intake. In one 1999 study, the researchers gave alcohol-preferring rats a salvia miltiorrhiza extract which led to a voluntary forty percent reduction in alcohol consumption by the animals. The investigators think the herb's ability to decrease alcohol absorption in the gastrointestinal tract was responsible for the reduction. A second and third experiment showed the salvia extract reduced the blood alcohol levels in the rats up to sixty percent compared to rats who were not given the extract. The researchers believe the decreased alcohol absorption did not result in the same "high" for the animals and they concluded herbs or drugs that reduce alcohol absorption in the body may be helpful to control drinking.

Another 2003 study from the same investigators found a standardized extract of salvia miltiorrhiza, IDN 5082, delayed alcohol drinking behavior in rats. The animals studied here had never experienced alcohol, even though they had been bred to be alcohol-preferring rats. Just before the animals were offered unlimited access to alcohol, they were given the extract once a day for ten days. IDN 5082 delayed alcohol drinking behavior in the rats, reduced their alcohol consumption and increased their water intake. More evidence to support the theory that dan shen or salvia miltiorrhiza may cut alcohol craving and intake.

The most recent study, also conducted in 2003 and coming from the same scientists, suggests IDN 5082 prevents an increase in alcohol consumption that occurs after an alcohol-free period. After seven days of abstinence, alcohol-preferring rats were given the extract and did not drink more alcohol than usual during the first hour they had access to it. Now if they would only start testing IDN 5082 on humans!

Side effects of dan shen may include skin rash, itching, indigestion and shortness of breath. The herb contains a substance which may cause drowsiness – do not drive or operate machinery if you take it. The remedy may affect blood clotting and may be unsafe for people taking drugs for cardiovascular disease. Avoid it if you are taking blood thinning, blood pressure, pain or anti-anxiety medication. Do not take this herb if you are pregnant or breastfeeding – it could cause bleeding and miscarriage. Consult your qualified Chinese practitioner or herbally-aware physician before considering dan shen, especially if you are taking any other herbs or medications or suffer from a pre-existing medical or psychological condition.

Ge Gen
Pueraria lobata

The Chinese have used ge gen to treat alcohol problems – hangovers, alcohol craving, alcohol intoxication and alcoholism – for thousands of years. Commonly known as kudzu, this wild plant grows in many Asian countries and in North America. Ge gen is a sweet, pungent, cool herb that works in the stomach and spleen meridians.

Chinese healers prescribe it to clear heat, reinvigorate yang and to relieve thirst – including the thirst for alcohol. Considered an anti-drunkenness herb, it is also recommended for fevers, headaches, diarrhea, aching muscles and convulsions.

Ge gen is rich in iron, calcium and phosphorous and contains two active ingredients, daidzin and daidzein. Modern research shows the remedy may increase blood supply to the brain, improve coronary circulation and prevent cardiovascular and liver damage. In addition to treating alcohol abuse, today it is also given for high blood pressure, angina pectoris, deafness, retinitis, allergies and dysentery.

David Lee, a chemist at the Research Triangle Institute in North Carolina, noticed many Chinese households keep an herbal tea mixture on hand which contains kudzu. Translated from Chinese, the name of the tea means "drunkenness dispeller." It has been used in China as a hangover cure and to reduce the effects of alcohol for centuries.

In 1992, Lee got together with David Overstreet and Amir Rezvani, associate research professors of psychiatry at the University of North Carolina at Chapel Hill Skipper Bowles Center for Alcohol Studies. They performed a number of experiments on rats who drank large quantities of alcohol and were administered the Chinese herbal compound. They noted the rats given the kudzu concoction drank less alcohol or drank normally. The scientists concluded if an herb, like kudzu, or a drug can slow down the alcohol metabolism process, alcohol remains in the system longer and less alcohol is needed. And decreased craving and consumption may be the result.

One 1992 study by Dr. Wing-Ming Keung and Dr. Bert Valle and colleagues at the Center for Biochemical and Biophysical Sciences and Medicine at Harvard Medical School in Boston, Massachusetts, showed the active ingredients of kudzu cut alcohol intake up to fifty percent in hamsters. And even though the extract significantly reduced alcohol consumption, it did not affect water or food intake by the animals.

In 1998, Dr. Scott Lukas, a pharmacologist at MacLean Hospital in Belmont, Massachusetts, reported the results of a study with human subjects who received a kudzu extract or a placebo, then were asked to down three shots of either vodka or a non-alcoholic drink in twenty minutes. Those who received the kudzu extract and drank the alcohol had lower blood alcohol levels and felt less drunk than those who took the placebo and drank the alcohol. Dr. Lukas believes kudzu may work in two different ways. First, it may reduce the alcohol that gets to the brain. Second, it may affect brain chemistry and reduce the positive feelings a person experiences when they drink alcohol. Dr. Lukas concluded if you do not achieve the high you expect when you drink alcohol, the less interest you will have in it.

Ge gen or kudzu may cause drowsiness – do not drive or operate machinery if you take it. Professional medical supervision is a must before you get serious about this remedy.

Ren Shen
Panax ginseng

Ren shen or ginseng has been a superstar in the Chinese pharmacy for over 2,000 years. It is a calming, mood-elevating and energy-boosting herb all rolled into one and it is prescribed for everything from indigestion to heart disease to cancer to stress to depression to alcoholism. In China, ren shen is offered as an anti-intoxicant and some recommend it as an antidote to alcohol craving. This sweet, bitter, warm herb affects the lung, heart, spleen, kidney and liver meridians.

Traditionally, it is given to increase qi, nourish the heart and quiet the spirit. It soothes the nervous system and is suggested for stress, anxiety, depression, restlessness, exhaustion, palpitations, insomnia and poor appetite. Digestive and heart problems are also treated with the remedy.

There are three types of ginseng: American and Asian ginseng, which belong to the same Panax species, and Siberian ginseng, which is a different plant altogether. The active ingredients in Asian and American ginseng are ginsenosides which are not contained in Siberian ginseng. However, all three are adaptogens. An adaptogen normalizes and strengthens body functions and protects you from physical and mental stress.

Even though all three ginsengs are adaptogens and may produce similar positive effects, American and Asian ginseng are the focus here because they contain ginsenosides which are responsible for most of the benefits associated with ginseng. American ginseng is the most popular ginseng used for medicinal purposes because it is milder and better suited for long-term use. But Asian ginseng is thought to be superior in treating alcohol abuse.

Physiologically, ginseng lowers blood pressure, regulates blood sugar, increases energy and physical stamina and maintains and protects the immune system. It is believed to speed up the breakdown of alcohol in the body and decrease alcohol absorption in the stomach.

Psychologically, ginseng reduces tension, anxiety and stress. Studies with human subjects revealed the remedy made them feel more tranquil, yet alert, compared to subjects given a placebo. Several animal studies concluded ginseng relieved stress as well as valium (a popular prescription tranquilizer), but without the negative side effects of valium. Other research suggests ginseng may help alleviate depression, alcoholism and attention-deficit disorder. It is also thought to stimulate the appetite and the sex life. A miracle medicine in anyone's book.

American ginseng is believed to be the most potent mood elevator. A study of 501 men and women found those taking ginseng reported increased feelings of well-being and personal satisfaction. They also enjoyed significant improvements in their energy level, sex life and sleep. American ginseng may help conquer alcohol craving because if you feel good physically and mentally, the less inclined you will be to alter your good mood with alcohol.

Even though some Chinese herbalists feel American ginseng is better for treating alcohol abuse because it is a cooling herb – cooling the fire and heat associated with alcohol abuse – others feel Asian ginseng is the most effective anti-craving agent. Human studies point to increased blood alcohol clearance with Asian ginseng. It appears to break down and clear alcohol from the body faster. And animal studies suggest it reduces alcohol absorption in the stomach. Some argue if you take Asian ginseng and do not achieve the "high" you expect from alcohol, because it is metabolized faster and not efficiently absorbed into the body, the less likely you are to crave alcohol.

Too much ginseng may cause headache, palpitations and agitation. Other side effects may include diarrhea, vomiting, high blood pressure, low blood sugar and insomnia. Do not take these herbs if you have high blood pressure, if you suffer from any gastrointestinal, heart or breast disease or if you are pregnant or breastfeeding. Do not take these remedies over a long period of time. Consult your physician before you consider taking Asian or American ginseng. They could exacerbate a pre-existing medical or psychological condition or interact with a number of medications, including antidepressant, anti-psychotic and blood-thinning medicines.

The Craving Game

Chinese herbal medicine is only one branch of traditional Chinese medicine. Some research shows acupuncture and acupressure may also reduce alcohol craving. Check out your local library for books on these subjects or talk to a licensed acupuncturist about treatments to decrease drinking desire and alcohol consumption. Start thinking outside of the box to tackle your alcohol appetite.

Chapter 10
Exotic Ayurvedic Cures
Reduce the Thirst for Alcohol

Ayurveda is one of the oldest medical systems in the world originating in India over 5,000 years ago. The word ayurveda comes from two Sanskrit words: "ayu" which means life and "veda" which means knowledge. Loosely translated, it means the "science of life." Ayurvedic herbs to remove impurities from the body, nurture the soul and reduce your thirst for alcohol are the focus of this chapter.

In Ayurveda, each person is a unique combination of body, mind and spiritual elements which make up their "constitution." A balance of these parts promotes wellness, while an imbalance of them causes disease. The goal of Ayurveda is to equalize these physical, mental and spiritual elements which will restore your original constitution and lead to good health. Herbal remedies are just one of many therapies an Ayurvedic practitioner may prescribe to help you achieve this goal.

What's your constitution? According to Ayurveda, your body is made up of five components – fire, earth, water, air and space or ether – and it is influenced by three energy forces or doshas – vata, kapha and pitta. Most often one dosha is dominant and another is secondary. Your dominant dosha determines your constitution.

Many Ayurvedic healers think addictive behaviors, like alcohol abuse, develop as a result of coping with and seeking relief from anxiety and fear and that each dosha deals with these feelings differently. The pitta personality, however, is most susceptible to problem drinking. If pitta is not in balance, anger, hatred and jealousy result and cause indigestion, hunger and thirst – including a thirst for alcohol. But balancing pitta with certain herbs may take the edge off of these negative emotions and alcohol appetite.

Even though there is little empirical evidence to support the use of many Ayurvedic medicines, believers feel Ayurveda would not have survived for so long if it didn't work. Note that Ayurvedic herbs are often combined with other herbs to reduce toxicity and increase effectiveness and each herb is known by Sanskrit, Hindi, English and botanical names. Sanskrit and botanical names are listed here.

Currently, the United States does not license Ayurvedic practitioners. If you pursue Ayurvedic treatment, best to take your interest to a qualified Ayurvedic professional or a physician who combines western medicine with Ayurvedic philosophy and therapies.

First, Heal and Rejuvenate Your Body

Amalaki
Emblica officinalis

Translated from Sanskrit, amalaki means "the sustainer." Commonly known as Indian gooseberry, it is considered one of the most powerful cleansing, renewing and anti-aging remedies in Ayurveda and it is thought to balance all three doshas – especially pitta.

Amalaki is prescribed to remove toxins from the blood and to restore and nourish the blood, liver, bones and skin. It is given for fevers, cough, diarrhea, dysentery, anemia, asthma, jaundice, respiratory problems and atherosclerosis. It is a popular medicine for infections and ulcers and is a prized anti-aging herb in India.

Amalaki fruit is very nutritious and contains the most concentrated natural vitamin C available. Only about one inch in diameter, it has as much ascorbic acid as two oranges plus minerals and amino acids. Possessing antioxidant, antibacterial and antiviral properties, amalaki purifies the blood and liver and protects the body from free radical damage. The herb also has a cooling, diuretic and laxative effect and initiates healing – helpful for anyone trying to cut down on alcohol.

Western medicine uses amalaki fruit to treat scurvy, gastritis and peptic ulcers. In one study, the remedy was given three times a day for seven days to twenty patients suffering from gastritis. It proved to be effective in eighty-five percent of the cases. This medicine has also been shown to reduce cholesterol and fatty tissue in the livers of animals. And other research with animals suggests the herb has heart-protecting qualities.

Amalaki is generally considered safe when properly prescribed. No information is available on the dangers or side effects of this remedy. Consult an Ayurvedic healer or your doctor if you are interested in this herb.

Bhringaraj
Eclipta alba

Grown throughout India, bhringaraj is a valued rejuvenating and anti-aging remedy in Ayurveda. Also known by the common name thistles, it is an important mind/body medicine – purifying the blood and liver and calming the spirit.

Ayurvedic practitioners prescribe it to reinvigorate pitta and to treat hepatitis, cirrhosis of the liver and enlarged spleen. The herb is also used for headaches, earaches and skin conditions. It is believed to improve liver and kidney functions, promote bone and tooth growth and sharpen eyesight and memory.

Bhringaraj is a strong antioxidant with antiviral and anti-inflammatory qualities. Two active ingredients, wedelolactone and dimethyl wedelolactone, are potent liver-protecting agents and help to restore the liver, kidneys and spleen. This remedy also stimulates the flow of bile and acts as a laxative.

Bhringaraj may cause severe chills. Supervision by a qualified Ayurvedic practitioner or your physician is a must before trying this herb.

Bhuamalaki
Phyllanthus niruri

For over 2,000 years bhuamalaki has been the most widely used Ayurvedic herb to treat liver problems. It is thought to pacify both pitta and kapha doshas and it is often used to treat liver diseases associated with alcohol abuse.

Traditionally, it is recommended for chronic alcohol-related liver diseases, including cirrhosis, viral hepatitis B and enlarged liver. Jaundice, diabetes, dysentery, skin sores and ulcers are also cared for with bhuamalaki. It is used to aid digestion, stimulate appetite and as a mild laxative as well.

The plant has antiviral, antiseptic and diuretic features. Although the active ingredient of this remedy is not known, it is considered to have liver-protecting properties. Studies show it blocks an enzyme required to replicate the hepatitis B virus.

This herb is considered safe when used correctly. No information is available on the toxicity or side effects of this remedy. Best to seek medical advice before considering bhuamalaki.

Bhunimba
Andrographis paniculata

Bhunimba is the main ingredient for a blood purifying tonic popular in India. This hardy plant is also known by the common names kalmegh and creat.

In Ayurveda, this herb is thought to restore and normalize body functions. It is given for digestive, spleen and liver disorders, including hepatitis. Fevers, flu, diarrhea and diabetes are also treated with bhunimba.

This remedy has antibacterial and laxative characteristics and andrographolide is the active ingredient responsible for its liver-protecting effect. Animal research from India indicates it prevents liver damage. And one Indian study showed ninety percent of human subjects given the herb for twenty-three days enjoyed significantly improved liver function.

Generally, this herb is considered safe when used as directed, but no information is available on side effects or dangers. Consult an Ayurvedic healer or your doctor before experimenting with this herb.

Ghee

Ghee is not an herb, but a miracle food and a mainstay in both the Indian kitchen and in Ayurvedic medicine. It is a cureall believed to promote vata and pitta balance, good health, well-being and long life. Melted butter with the milk solids and lactose removed, it does not contain hydrogenated oils or "bad" fat. It only contains the "good" fat essential for robust health.

Rich, buttery ghee has been used for thousands of years for everything from sinus problems to depression to rashes, headaches, diarrhea and allergies. Ancient Ayurvedic writings claim it aids digestion by balancing stomach acid and repairing and maintaining the lining of the stomach. This ultimate cooking oil also helps with the body's absorption of vitamins and minerals and it is often combined with other herbs because it helps them to penetrate the intestinal wall. Ghee is also applied as a topical ointment for skin conditions, including burns – preventing blistering and scarring. And nose drops of the oil are thought to clean the sinuses and improve voice and eyesight. It's a favorite anti-aging remedy and many think it enhances memory, learning and mental functioning.

Ghee is considered safe. No information is available on the side effects or toxicity of this remedy.

Haridra
Curcuma longa

Haridra is another powerful detoxifying herb prescribed in Ayurveda. Also known as the spice turmeric, it's a great excuse to feast on Indian food because it's used in so many of the dishes.

Ayurvedic practitioners suggest this remedy to cleanse the blood and body. It is given for liver and gallbladder problems, diabetes, acne, allergies and rashes. It is also offered to aid digestion and to strengthen the liver and immune system. Haridra is thought to improve the complexion.

This spice has anti-inflammatory, antioxidant, antibacterial and antiseptic qualities. It contains iron and potassium and the active ingredient is curcumin. Curcumin is a strong antioxidant – fighting free radicals that cause disease. Laboratory and animal studies show turmeric has detoxifying and liver-protecting characteristics. It increases an enzyme which facilitates the removal of toxins from the body and shields the liver from a number of dangerous substances, including acetaminophen and tetrachloride. Turmeric has also been shown to balance and prevent the oxidation of cholesterol and reduce the inflammation of brain cells which causes Alzheimer's disease.

Haridra is considered safe when used as recommended. No information is available on the dangers or side effects of this remedy.

Haritaki
Terminalia chebula

Loosely translated from Sanskrit, haritaki means "takes away disease." Found throughout India, this herb is famous for its anti-stress and anti-aging benefits.

In Ayurveda, it is given to clean and nourish the blood and body tissues and relieve digestive, heart and skin conditions. Coughs, asthma, anemia, vomiting, diarrhea, fever, liver and spleen disorders are also treated with the herb. Haritaki is believed to promote healthy skin, eyes and liver.

The plant is an adaptogen with liver-protecting properties. The active ingredients are chebulagic, chebulinic acid and corilagin.

Haritaki is not recommended if you are pregnant or suffering from exhaustion or dehydration. The toxicity and side effects of this remedy have not been thoroughly researched. Supervision by a qualified Ayurvedic professional or your physician is required before testing this herb.

Kutki
Picorrhiza kurroa

In India, kutki has been a cure for indigestion for centuries. It is considered a potent liver and gallbladder cleanser and it grows in the western Himalayas.

Traditional healers treat a number of different health problems, from asthma to snake bites to arthritis to liver disease, including the hepatitis B virus, with kutki. It is also given for fevers, constipation, skin diseases and epilepsy. The herb is thought to improve eyesight.

Kutki has anti-inflammatory and liver-protecting characteristics. The active ingredients are glycosides. The remedy repairs and rejuvenates liver cells and strengthens the immune system. Animal studies show it guards the liver by controlling abnormal changes in the cells. Other research concluded it protects animals from dangerous liver toxins as well or better than milk thistle and it actually reduces the formation of liver cancer cells caused by chemical exposures. Human studies suggest it may also be helpful in treating asthma and arthritis.

The safety of this plant has not been investigated. Side effects may include diarrhea and colic. Do not take this herb if you are pregnant or breastfeeding. Take your interest in kutki to a qualified Ayurvedic practitioner or your doctor.

Nimba
Azadirachta indica

Nimba is believed to be one of the finest detoxifying, immune-system boosting remedies available in Ayurvedic medicine. Native to India and Iran, this herb is an excellent blood purifier and is currently being examined as a treatment for cancer and AIDS.

Many consider nimba a cureall. Dozens of ailments, including fevers, headache, sore throat, colds, flu, diabetes, arthritis and blood, skin, kidney, liver and heart disorders, are treated with the remedy. It is also prescribed for nerve and digestive problems, bruises and wounds, malaria, sexually-transmitted diseases, mononucleosis and yeast and fungal infections.

Nimba offers antibacterial, antiviral, anti-inflammatory, antiseptic, antioxidant and anti-cancer benefits. It lowers blood pressure, blood sugar and heart cholesterol levels. An effective treatment for diabetes, it reduces the need for insulin up to fifty percent. The herb has also been shown to reduce anxiety and enhance feelings of well-being.

Long term use of nimba is not recommended unless it is combined with other herbs or mixed with honey or butter. The side effects and dangers of this remedy are not known. If you are serious about nimba, consult a qualified Ayurvedic healer or your physician.

Next, Heal and Rejuvenate Your Mind

Ashvaganda
Withania somnifera

The Sanskrit name for this evergreen shrub translates as "smelling like a horse" – implying you will feel the strength of a horse when you eat it. Also known as Indian ginseng, this soothing herb is believed to promote vitality and long life.

Ashvaganda is given for mind and body stress. It calms and nourishes the nervous system, balances the mood and some practitioners use it to treat alcoholism. Arthritis, rheumatism, hypertension, asthma, diabetes and nervous exhaustion are also cared for with the remedy. It's considered an aphrodisiac and a sleeping aid as well.

Ashvaganda is an adaptogen with sedative, antioxidant and diuretic properties. The active ingredients are withanolides which are similar to the active ingredients in Asian ginseng. In addition to having a calming effect, animal studies show it also has liver-protecting qualities and it increases physiological endurance.

Do not take this remedy if you take tranquilizers or anticonvulsants or if you are pregnant or breastfeeding. It should be avoided if you have a cold or the flu. Medical supervision is a must before considering ashvaganda.

Brahmi
Bacopa monniera

In Sanskrit, brahmi means "Goddess of Supreme Wisdom" because it is thought this herb paves the way to wisdom. It is one of the most highly regarded revitalizing herbs in Ayurveda – nurturing the body and mind and relaxing yet reinvigorating the nervous system. And even though it is considered a weed in India, many believe this bitter, cool remedy imparts profound mental benefits.

Brahmi is a tranquilizing herb which also increases energy and improves memory, concentration, learning ability and intellect. It is prescribed to relieve anxiety, stress and depression and to encourage mental balance and clarity. The remedy is thought to cleanse the blood, liver, nerves and brain and it is also used to treat fevers, joint pain, skin conditions, asthma, mental illness and epilepsy. Brahmi is often recommended for cognitive problems associated with aging.

This herb has antibacterial, antioxidant and antifungal features. The active ingredients are alkaloids and saponins which produce a calming, antidepressant effect. Considered "brain food", brahmi stimulates protein synthesis in brain cells resulting in enhanced memory, intelligence and mental acuity. It has also been shown to promote circulation, lower high blood pressure and increase blood sugar levels. Today, it is also used to treat hepatitis, cancer, memory loss, attention-deficit disorder and hyperactivity.

Brahmi is considered safe when properly prescribed. No information is available on the side effects or dangers of this remedy. Seek the advice of an Ayurvedic practitioner or your physician before trying this herb.

Mandukaparni
Centella asiatica

Mandukaparni is another spiritual, revitalizing remedy in the Ayurvedic pharmacy. Commonly known as gotu kola, it clears impurities from blood, liver and brain cells, quiets negative emotions and has a calming yet energizing effect.

Used in Ayurveda to "balance the brain", it is thought to tranquilize and reinvigorate the nerves and the brain. It is prescribed for mental and physical fatigue, to raise energy levels and to improve meditation. The herb is also used to treat high blood pressure, skin diseases, cancer, arthritis and hepatitis. It encourages sleep and strengthens the immune system.

This remedy contains calcium, magnesium and vitamin K and there are three active ingredients which account for its versatility. One is an antibiotic which helps healing. Another is an anti-inflammatory which reduces swelling. And a third which produces a sedative effect.

Mandukaparni aids in tissue development – cutting healing time and scar tissue and promoting healthy skin, hair and nails. It improves circulation throughout the body and test tube studies show it destroys cultured tumor cells. The herb is not only healing and nourishing, but stimulating too. It sharpens mental functioning, concentration and memory and has been shown to increase IQ levels and decrease behavioral problems in mentally retarded children.

Mandukaparni is generally considered safe when used as recommended. The side effects and toxicity of this remedy are not known so it is best to consult with an Ayurvedic professional or your doctor before experimenting with this herb.

Shankhapushpi
Convolvulus microphyllus

An important tranquilizer, shankhapushpi is believed to not only lessen mental tension, but to better memory, learning and recall. Also known as bindweed, the plant grows in northern India.

Traditionally, it is recommended to reduce stress and restlessness. Nervous system, skin and mental problems, neuralgia and rheumatism are all treated with shankhapushpi. The herb is also prescribed for insomnia.

Alkaloids are the principal ingredients of the plant. Clinical trials with patients suffering from arterial hypertension showed a drop in blood pressure when they were given the remedy. It is also thought to rejuvenate nerve tissue and bone marrow and lower cholesterol. Animal studies show a reduction in total serum cholesterol after being treated with the herb for thirty days.

Shankhapushpi is considered safe when used as directed. However, the side effects and dangers of this remedy have not been thoroughly investigated. Take your interest in this herb to an Ayurvedic healer or your physician.

Finally, Reduce Your Thirst for Alcohol

Punarnava
Boerrhavia diffusa

One of the few Ayurvedic herbs prescribed for alcohol abuse, punarnava is commonly known as spreading hogweed. Two varieties of hogweed exist – red and white – the red variety is credited with relieving chronic alcoholism.

In addition to alcohol abuse, Ayurvedic practitioners give it for liver, gallbladder and kidney ailments. Heart and skin diseases, rheumatism, asthma, jaundice and insomnia are also cared for with this remedy. Many believe it promotes long life.

Punarnava has pain-killing, laxative, diuretic and anti-convulsant properties. Even though some recommend it to reduce alcohol craving and consumption, no research supporting this use has been conducted to date.

Little information on the safety or side effects of punarnava is available. Large doses of the herb may cause vomiting. Consult an Ayurvedic professional or your doctor before testing punarnava.

SKV

SKV is an herbal formula which has been shown to lower voluntary alcohol consumption in animals. It is brewed from fermented sugar cane and raisins plus twelve other herbal ingredients.

Research conducted by E. R. Shanmugasundaram and colleagues at the University of Madras in India showed rats with access to alcohol who were given the herbal formula significantly reduced their alcohol intake. SKV also appeared to reduce fatty deposits in the liver. Another study by the same scientists indicated animals given the formula not only lowered their alcohol consumption, but increased their food intake. And a third animal study by the Indian investigators showed SKV not only cut drinking, but decreased both the blood alcohol levels with no withdrawal symptoms and the organ enlargement associated with alcohol abuse.

No attention has been paid to this herbal formula since these early studies. The next step is to conduct human trials with SKV. Information on the side effects or dangers of this medicine is not available. Seek your doctor's advice if you entertain the thought of SKV.

Vacha
Acorus calamus

Vacha is believed to be a brain and nervous system rejuvenator and has been prescribed to curb alcohol craving by some Ayurvedic healers. Grown throughout India, it is also considered an aphrodisiac and is frequently referred to as "natural Viagra." Commonly known as calamus, it is also used in European and Native American herbal medicine.

Vacha is used as a sedative and to relieve fever, asthma and bronchitis. It is thought to promote cerebral circulation and it is given to treat symptoms associated with the head and brain, including epilepsy and neuralgia. Mental disorders, dysentery, liver and kidney problems are all cared for with this remedy. Even though some practitioners recommend it as an anti-alcohol craving agent, there is no scientific evidence to support this use.

The United States Food and Drug Administration contends this herb is "not intended for human consumption" because large doses of isolated ingredients of the plant given to rats over a long period of time proved to be carcinogenic. Vacha could be hazardous to your health and should be taken only under the supervision of a qualified Ayurvedic professional or your physician.

The Craving Game

What's your constitutional type? Pick up a book on Ayurvedic medicine or consult an Ayurvedic practitioner and find out. Next, look into pancha karma, a detoxification and purification ritual which eliminates impurities produced by an imbalance of the three doshas. Then turn your attention to yoga and aromatherapy. Which of these treatments could help you reduce your alcohol craving and consumption?

Part Five:
FOR MORE INFORMATION . . .

About the Author,
Donna J. Cornett, M.A.

Donna J. Cornett is the founder and director of Drink/Link Moderate Drinking Programs and Products. She holds an M.A. and California College Teaching Credential in psychology and is a member of the American Psychological Association. She believes offering drinkers a moderate drinking goal, instead of life-long abstinence, is the key to motivating drinkers to seek early treatment and to preventing alcohol abuse.

Cornett was in her thirties when she realized she was drinking too much and would be facing a serious drinking problem if she did not address it immediately. At that time her only options were abstinence, AA or to keep on drinking. There was no middle-of-the-road alcohol education program teaching drinkers sensible drinking habits and attitudes so they could avoid alcohol abuse. But like many drinkers, she did not believe her drinking was serious enough to stop altogether or in the concept of a "higher power" to help her cut down.

Consequently, Cornett developed Drink/Link in 1988 – long before any other moderate drinking programs were available in the United States. This commonsense program teaches drinkers the art of moderate drinking and prevents alcoholism.

Donna J. Cornett is also the author of *7 Weeks to Safe Social Drinking: How to Effectively Moderate Your Alcohol Intake* and the motivational audiotape "Control Your Drinking – Now!". She has been featured or consulted for articles in Time Magazine, the New York Post, ABC News.com, Scripps Howard News Service and professional publications. Her latest achievement is offering drinkers everywhere the first affordable, over-the-counter alcohol abuse prevention program – The Sensible Drinking System.

To contact Donna Cornett email her at info@drinklinkmoderation.com, call her at 707-539-5465 or write her at P.O. Box 5441, Santa Rosa, California, USA, 95402.

About Drink/Link™
Moderate Drinking Programs & Products

Drink/Link Moderate Drinking Programs and Products was established in 1988 and has helped thousands of drinkers worldwide to modify drinking habits and attitudes, reduce alcohol consumption and prevent alcoholism. Drink/Link was the first moderate drinking program in the United States and the first registered with both the California Department of Alcohol and Drug Programs and the U.S. Department of Health and Human Services.

All Drink/Link Programs are based on commonsense safe-drinking guidelines and clinically-proven behavioral, cognitive, motivational and lifestyle strategies and techniques to help you stay within those guidelines. The most intensive programs, which include professional counseling, are the Email Counseling Program and the Telephone Counseling Program. The Self-Study Program and the Sensible Drinking System are self-help programs which you complete on your own at home.

Drink/Link also offers a complete line of moderate drinking products. A workbook, *7 Weeks to Safe Social Drinking: How to Effectively Moderate Your Alcohol Intake* by Donna J. Cornett, a motivational audiotape, "Control Your Drinking – Now!" by Donna J. Cornett, Nutritional and Moderation Supplements to reduce alcohol craving, a Drinking Diary, a Drink Graph and a Breath Analyzer to keep you on the moderate drinking track.

"Drink/Link Moderate Drinking Tips" – a monthly newsletter – discusses the latest research on moderate drinking and alcohol abuse as

147

well as complementary and alternative medicine tips and treatments to control alcohol craving and consumption. Thinking outside of the box to encourage safe drinking and prevent alcohol abuse is what this newsletter is all about. Email us to get on the mailing list today.

Contact Drink/Link directly at www.ModerateDrinkingPrograms.com to view the product catalog or call us toll-free at 888-773-7465 to order a product. Or contact the nearest retail outlet that carries Drink/Link products.

Drink/Link™

MODERATE DRINKING PROGRAMS & PRODUCTS

ORDER FORMS

Order Your Own Copy of

7 Weeks to Safe Social Drinking:
How to Effectively Moderate Your Alcohol Intake
by Donna J. Cornett

NUMBER OF BOOKS _____

COST OF BOOKS _____
(Paperback-$18.95)

OUTSIDE USA
      ADD 10% _____

SHIPPING & HANDLING _____
(U.S.: $4.00 for first book &
$2.00 for each additional
book. Outside U.S.: $6.00
for first book & $4.00 for
each additional book.
Shipped U.S. Mail)

SUBTOTAL _____

STATE TAX _____
(California residents please add tax)

FINAL TOTAL* _____
*Prices are in U.S. dollars and may be subject to change.

PAYMENT ENCLOSED $_____

PLEASE CHARGE TO MY
CREDIT CARD:
(Visa, MasterCard,
American Express,
Discover, ATM
Bankcards Accepted)

Account #_____

Expiration Date _____

Signature _____

PLEASE SEND TO:

NAME _____

INSTITUTION _____

ADDRESS _____

CITY _____

STATE/ZIP _____

COUNTRY _____

TELEPHONE _____ EMAIL_____

May we use your email address for order confirmation and other information? Yes No

Order Directly or From Your Local Bookstore

Drink/Link ™
MODERATE DRINKING PROGRAMS & PRODUCTS
P.O. BOX 5441
SANTA ROSA, CALIFORNIA USA 95402
TELEPHONE: 707-539-5465   TOLL-FREE: 888-773-7465
FAX: 707-537-1010
EMAIL: info@drinklinkmoderation.com
www.ModerateDrinkingPrograms.com
www.drinklinkmoderation.com

Drink/Link ™
MODERATE DRINKING PROGRAMS & PRODUCTS
ORDER FORM

FOR A COMPLETE LISTING OF PROGRAMS & PRODUCTS LOGON TO:

www.ModerateDrinkingPrograms.com
www.drinklinkmoderation.com
Toll-Free: 888-773-7465
Local: 707-539-5465
Fax: 707-537-1010

The *Drink/Link* ™ Self-Study Program – $195*

This program includes the workbook, *7 Weeks to Safe Social Drinking*, the motivational audiotape, "Control Your Drinking – Now!", the Herbal and All-Natural Tips Booklet, a Drinking Diary, Drink Graph, Nutritional Supplements and Step-by-Step Instructions so you can successfully complete the program on your own at home. It also includes a 50-minute telephone consultation with Donna Cornett – examining your current drinking habits and offering tips tailored to your lifestyle so you drink less.

The *Drink/Link* ™ Sensible Drinking System $79.99*

This over-the-counter program includes the basics – the workbook, *7 Weeks to Safe Social Drinking*, the motivational audiotape, "Control Your Drinking – Now!", a Drinking Diary, Drink Graph and Step-by-Step Instructions so you can successfully complete the program on your own at home.

*Prices are in U.S. dollars and may be subject to change.

PLEASE CIRCLE THE PROGRAM OF CHOICE:

The *Drink/Link*™ **Self Study Program – $195**

The *Drink/Link*™ **Sensible Drinking System $79.99**

NUMBER OF PROGRAMS _____   PAYMENT ENCLOSED $_____

COST OF PROGRAMS _____   PLEASE CHARGE TO
                                   MY CREDIT CARD:
OUTSIDE USA   (Visa, MasterCard,
        ADD 10% _____   American Express,
                                   Discover, ATM
                                   Bankcard Accepted)

                                   Account # _____

SHIPPING & HANDLING _____
(U.S.: $10.00 for first program.   Expiration Date _____
Outside U.S.: $15.00 for first
& $10.00 for each additional   Signature _____
program. Shipped U.S. Mail)

SUBTOTAL _____

STATE TAX _____
(California residents
please add tax)

FINAL TOTAL _____

PLEASE SEND TO:

NAME_____

INSTITUTION _____

ADDRESS _____

CITY _____

STATE/ZIP _____

COUNTRY _____

TELEPHONE_____ EMAIL _____

May we use your email address for order confirmation and other information? Yes   No

Drink/Link ™
MODERATE DRINKING PROGRAMS & PRODUCTS
P.O. BOX 5441
SANTA ROSA, CALIFORNIA USA 95402
TELEPHONE: 707-539-5465   TOLL-FREE: 888-773-7465
FAX: 707-537-1010
EMAIL: info@drinklinkmoderation.com
www.ModerateDrinkingPrograms.com
www.drinklinkmoderation.com

BIBLIOGRAPHY

American Psychiatric Association. *Diagnostic and Statistical Manual of Mental Disorders, 4th ed., rev.* Washington, D.C.: American Psychiatric Association, 1994.

Anton, R. F. "Obsessive-compulsive aspects of craving: development of the Obsessive Compulsive Drinking Scale." *Addiction* 95(2): S211-S217, 2000.

Anton, R. F. "What is Craving?" *Alcohol Research & Health* 23(3), 1999.

Arase, Y, et al. "The long term efficacy of glycyrrhizin in chronic hepatitis C patients." *Cancer* 79(8): 1494-500, 1997.

Astin, J. A. "Why patients use alternative medicine: results of a national study." *Journal of the American Medical Association* 279:1548-53, 1998.

Atkins, R. C. *Dr. Atkin's Nutrition Breakthrough.* New York: Smithmark Publishing, 1984.

Atkins, R. C. *Dr. Atkin's Vita-Nutrient Solution.* New York: Simon and Schuster, 1998.

Baker, H. "A vitamin profile of alcoholism." *International Journal of Vitamin and Nutritional Research* 24:179, 1983.

Balch, J. F., and P. A. Balch. *Prescription for Nutritional Healing, 2nd ed.* Garden City Park, NY: Avery Publishing Group, 1997.

Beckmann, H., D. Athen, M. Olteanu, and R. Zimmer. "DL-phenylalanine versus imipramine: a double-blind controlled study." *Archiv fur Psychiatrie und Nervenkrankheiten* 227:49-58, 1979.

Bellenir, K. *Alcoholism Sourcebook.* Detroit: Omnigraphics, Inc., 2000.

Bensky, D., and A. Gamble. *Chinese Herbal Medicine: Materia Medica, rev. ed.* Seattle: Eastland Press, 1993.

Biery, J. R., J. H. Williford, and E. A. McMullen. "Alcohol craving in rehabilitation: assessment of nutrition therapy." *Journal of the American Dietetic Association* 91:463-6, 1991.

Blum, K. "A commentary on neurotransmitter restoration as a common mode of treatment for alcohol, cocaine and opiate abuse." *Integrative Psychiatry* 6:199-204, 1986.

Blum, K., and J. E. Payne. *Alcohol and the Addictive Brain.* New York: Macmillan, 1991.

Blum, K., C. Reuben., D. Gastelu, and D. K. Miller. "Nutritional Gene Therapy: Natural Healing in Recovery." *Counselor Magazine* February, 2001.

Blumenthal, M., W. Busse, A. Goldberg., eds., et al. *The Complete German Commission E Monographs.* Boston: Integrative Medicine Communications, 1998.

Blumenthal, M., A. Goldberg, and J. Brinckmann. *Herbal Medicine: Expanded Commission E Monographs.* Newton, MA: Integrative Medicine Communications, 2000.

Boericke, W. *Pocket Book Manual of Homeopathic Materia Medica, 9th ed.* St. Louis, MO: Formur International, 1982.

Bourin, M., T. Bougerol, G. Guitton, et al. "A combination of plant extracts in the treatment of outpatients with adjustment disorder with anxious mood: controlled study versus placebo." *Fundamental and Clinical Pharmacology* 11:127-132, 1997.

Brunetti, G., S. Serr, G. Vacca, C. Lobin, P. Morazzoni, E. Bombardelli, G. Colombo, L. Gessa, and M. A. Carai. "IDN 5082, a standardized extract of Salvia miltiorrhiza, delays acquisition of alcohol drinking behavior in rats." *Journal of Ethnopharmacology* 85(1):93-7, 2003.

Buimovici-Klein, E., V. Mohan, M. Lange, et al. "Inhibition of HIV replication in lymphocyte cultures of virus-positive subjects in the presence of sho-saiko-to, an oriental plant extract." *Antiviral Research* 14: 279-86, 1990.

Bullock, M. L., P. D. Culliton, and R. T. Olander. "Controlled trial of acupuncture for severe recidivist alcoholism." *Lancet* 24:1(8652):1435-9, 1989.

Bullock, M. L., A. J. Umen, and P. D. Culliton. "Acupuncture treatment of alcoholic recidivism: a pilot study." *Alcoholism Clinical and Experimental Research* 11(3):292-5, 1987.

Burnett, J. C. *Gout and its Cure.* New Delhi: B. Jain Publisher, 1998.

Carai, M. A. M., R. Agabio, E. Bombardelli, et al. "Potential use of medicinal plants in the treatment of alcoholism." *Fitotherapy* 71:S38-S42, 2000.

Caso Marasco, A., R. Vargas Ruiz, A. Salas Villagomez, and C. Begon Infante. "Double-blind study of multivitamin complex supplemented with ginseng extract." *Drug Experimental and Clinical Research* 22(6):323-329, 1996.

Clarke, J. H. *A Dictionary of Practical Materia Medica.* Essex, UK: S.W. Daniel Co. Ltd., 1991.

Cleary, J. P. "Etiology and biological treatment of alcohol addiction." *Journal of Neurological and Orthopaedic Medicine and Surgery* 6:75-77, 1985.

Cleary, J. P. "Niacinimide and addictions." *Journal of Nutritional Medicine* 1:83-84, 1990.

Colombo, G., R. Agabio, C. Lobina, R. Reali, P. Morazzoni, E. Bombardelli, and G. L. Gessa. "Salvia miltiorrhiza extract inhibits alcohol absorption, preference and discrimination in sP rats." *Alcohol* 18(1):65-70, 1999.

Corbett, R., J. F. Menez, H. H. Flock, and B. E. Leonard. "The effects of chronic ethanol administration on rat liver and erythrocyte lipid composition: modulatory role of evening primrose oil." *Alcohol Alcoholism* 26(4):459-464, 1991.

Deak, G., et al. "Immunomodulator effect of silymarin therapy in chronic alcoholic liver diseases." *Orvosi Hetilap* 130(51):2723-7, 1989.

De Smet, P. A. G., and W. Nolen. "St. John's Wort as an antidepressant." *British Medical Journal* 313:241-242, 1996.

Ellis, F. R., and S. A. Nasser. "Pilot study of viamin B12 in the treatment of tiredness." *British Journal of Nutrition* 30:277-83, 1973.

Erdmann, R., and M. Jones. *The Amino Revolution.* New York: McGraw-Hill, 1987.

Eriksson, C. .J. "Increase in hepatic NAD level – its effect on the detox state and on ethanol and acetaldehyde metabolism." *Federation of Europe Biochemical Society* 40:3117-20, 1974.

Eriksson, K., L. Pekkanen, and M. Rusi. "The effects of dietary thiamin on voluntary ethanol drinking and ethanol metabolism in the rat." *British Journal of Nutrition* 43(1):1-13, 1980.

Ferenci, P., B. Dragosics, H. Dittrich, et al. "Randomized controlled trial of silymarin treatment in patients with cirrhosis of the liver." *Journal of Hepatology* 9:105-113, 1989.

Foster, S., and V. Tyler. *Tyler's Honest Herbal, 4th ed.* Binghamton, NY: Haworth Press, 1999.

Frawley, D. *Ayurvedic Healing: A Comprehensive Guide.* Twin Lakes, WI: Lotus Press 2000.

Gach, M. R. *Acupressure's Potent Points.* New York: Bantam, 1990.

Gibo, Y., Y. Nakamura, N. Takahashi, et al. "Clinical study of sho-saiko-to therapy for japanese patients with chronic hepatitis C (CH-C)." *Progressive Medicine* 14:217-19, 1994.

Griffith, H. W. *Vitamins, Herbs, Minerals & Supplements: The Complete Guide, rev.ed.* Tucson, AZ.: Fisher Books, 1998.

Guenther, R. M. "Role of nutritional therapy in alcoholism treatment." *International Journal of Biosocial Research* 4:5-18, 1983.

Handa, S. S., and A. Sharma. "Hepatoprotective effects of Andrographis paniculata against carbon tetrachloride-induced liver damage." *Indian Journal of Medical Research* 92:276-83, 1990.

Harrer, G., and V. Schulz. "Clinical investigation of the antidepressant effectiveness of hypericum." *Journal of Geriatric Psychiatry and Neurology* 7(1):56-8, 1994.

Hendler, S. S. *The Doctor's Vitamin and Mineral Encyclopedia.* New York: Simon & Schuster, 1990.

Hirayama, C., M. Okumura, K. Tankikawa, et al. "A multicenter randomized controlled clinical trial of sho-saiko-to in chronic active hepatitis." *Gastroenterologia Japonica* 24:715-19, 1989.

Hong, Y. H. *Oriental Materia Medica: A Concise Guide.* Long Beach, CA: Oriental Healing Arts Institute, 1986.

Horrobin, D. F. "A biochemical basis for alcoholism and alcohol-induced damage including fetal alcohol syndrome and cirrhosis: interference with essential fatty acid and prostaglandin metabolism." *Medical Hypotheses* 9:929-942, 1980.

Hulman, D. *The Consumer's Guide to Homeopathy.* New York: Tarcher/Putnam, 1995.

Jellinek, E. M., H. Isbell, G. Lundquist, H. M. Tiebout, H. Duchene, J. Maredones, and I. D. Macleod. "The 'craving' for alcohol." *Quarterly Journal of Studies on Alcohol* 16:34-66, 1955.

Jonas, W. B., and J. Jacobs. *Healing with Homeopathy.* New York: Warner Books, 1996.

Kelly, G. S. "Nutritional and botanical interventions to assist with the adaptation to stress." *Alternative Medicine Review* 4(4):249-265, 1999.

Keung, W. M., and B. L. Vallee. "Daidzin and daidzein suppress free-choice ethanol intake by Syrian golden hamsters." *Proceedings of the National Academy of Sciences USA* 90(21):10008-12, 1993.

Keung, W. M., and B. L. Vallee. "Kudzu root: an ancient Chinese source of modern antidipsotropic agents." *Phytochemistry* 47(4):499-506, 1998.

Keung, W. M., and B. L. Valle. "Therapeutic lessons from traditional Oriental medicine to contemporary Occidental pharmacology." *Experientia Supplementa* 71: 371-81, 1994.

Kinzler, E., J. Kromer, and E. Lehmann. "Clinical efficacy of a kava extract in patients with anxiety syndrome: double-blind placebo controlled study over 4 weeks." *Arzneimittel Forschung* 41:584-8, 1991.

Kleijnen, J., P. Knipschild, and G. Ter Riet. "Clinical trials of homeopathy." *British Medical Journal* 302:316-23, 1991.

Lad, V. *The Complete Book of Ayurvedic Home Remedies.* New York: Three Rivers Press, 1998.

Leathwood, P. D., et al. "Aqueous extract of valerian root improves sleep quality in man." *Pharmacology Biochemistry and Behavior* 17(1):65-71, 1982.

Lee, F. C., J. H. Ko, J. K. Park, and J. S. Lee. "Effects of Panax ginseng on blood alcohol clearance in man." *Clinical and Experimental Pharmacology and Physiology* 14(6): 543-6, 1987.

Li, X. Y. "Bioactivity of neolignans from fructus Schizandrae." *Memorias do Instituto Oswaldo Cruz.* 86:31-37, 1991.

Li, X. J., B. L. Zhao, G. T. Liu, and W. J. Xin. "Scavenging effects on active oxygen radicals by schizandrins with different structures and configurations." *Free Radical Biology and Medicine* 9:99-104, 1990.

Lin, R. C., S. Guthrie, C. Y. Xie, K. Mai, K. Y. Lee, L. Lumeng, and T. K. Li. "Isoflavonoid compounds extracted from Pueraria lobata suppress alcohol preference in pharmacogenetic rat model of alcoholism." *Alcoholism Clinical and Experimental Research* 20(4):659-63, 1996.

Lindahl, O., and L. Lindwall. "Double blind study of valerian preparation." *Pharmacology Biochemistry and Behavior* 32:1065-66, 1989.

Linde, K., R. Ramirez, et al. "Are the clinical effects of homeopathy placebo effects? A meta-analysis of placebo-controlled trials." *Lancet* 250:834-43, 1997.

Linde, K., G. Ramirez, C. D. Mulrow, et al. "St. John's wort for depression: an overview and meta-analysis." *British Medical Journal* 313:253-58, 1996.

Lindenbaum J., E. B. Healton, D. G. Savage, et al. "Neuropsychiatric disorders caused by cobalamin deficiency in the absence of anemia or macrocytosis." *New England Journal of Medicine* 318:1720-8, 1988.

Liu, G. T. "Pharmacological actions and clinical use of fructus Schizandrae." *Chinese Medical Journal* 102:740-749, 1989.

Liu, K. T. "Studies on fructus Schizandrae chinensis." Plenary lecture, World Health Organization Seminar on the Use of Medicinal Plants in

Health Care, Tokyo, September 1977. In *WHO Regional Office for the Western Pacific, Final Report.* Manila 101-12, 1997.

L'Orange, D. *Herbal Healing Secrets of the Orient.* Paramus, NJ: Prentice Hall, 1998.

Ludwig, A. *Understanding the Alcoholic's Mind.* New York: Oxford University Press, 1988.

Malesky, G. and the Editors of Prevention Health Books. *Nature's Medicine.* Emmaus, PA: Rodale Press, 1999.

Malhotra, S. C., ed. "Pharmacological investigations of certain medicinal plants and compound formulas used in Ayurveda and Siddha." *Central Council for Research in Ayurveda and Siddha* New Delhi, India, 1996.

Markowitz, J. S. "Herbal medicines assuming a larger role in psychiatric care." *Drug Topics* 142(17): 50-51, 1998.

Marlatt, G. A. "Craving for alcohol, loss of control, and relapse: A cognitive-behavioral analysis," in Nathan, P. E., G. A. Marlatt, and T. Loberg, eds. *Alcoholism: New Directions in Behavioral Research and Treatment.* New York: Plenum Press, 1978.

Marlatt, G. A., and J. R. Gordon. "Determinants of relapse: Implications of the maintenance of behavior change," in Davidson, P. O., and S. M. Davidson, eds. *Behavioral Medicine: Changing Health Lifestyle.* New York: Brunner/Mazel, 1980.

Marlatt, G. A., and J. R. Gordon, eds. *Relapse Prevention: Maintenance Strategies in the Treatment of Addictive Behaviors.* New York: Guilford Press, 1985.

McCabe, V. *Practical Homeopathy.* New York: St. Martin's Griffin, 2000.

McCaleb, R. "Valerian: nature's potent sleep aid." *Better Nutrition for Today's Living* 52(8):20- 23, 1990.

Monte, T. *World Medicine: The East West Guide to Healing Your Body.* New York: Putnam Publishing Group, 1993.

Monti, P. M., et al. "Cue exposure with coping skills treatment for male alcoholics: a preliminary investigation." *Journal of Consulting and Clinical Psychology* 61:1011-1019, 1993.

Monti, P., J. A. Binkoff, D. B. Abrams, W. R. Zwick, T. D. Nirenberg, and M. R. Liepman. "Reactivity of alcoholics and nonalcoholics to drinking cues." *Journal of Abnormal Psychology* 96:122-126, 1987.

Morazzoni, F., and E. Bombardelli. "Hypericum perforatum." *Fitoterapia* 66:43-68, 1995.

Mose, L. "Medicine for stress behind the wheel?" *Deutsche Apotheker Zeitung* 121:2651-4, 1981.

Murray, M., and J. Pizzorno. *Encyclopedia of Natural Medicine, 2nd ed., rev.* Rocklin, CA: Prima Health, 1998.

National Center for Complementary and Alternative Medicine. *"About the National Center for Complementary and Alternative Medicine."* www.nccam.nih.gov, 2004.

National Institute on Alcohol Abuse and Alcoholism. *10th Special Report to the U. S. Congress on Alcohol and Health.* Washington D. C.: U. S. Department of Health and Human Services, 2000.

National Institute on Alcohol Abuse and Alcoholism. *"Alcohol Alert-Craving Research: Implications for Treatment."* www.niaaa.nih.gov, 2001.

National Institute on Alcohol Abuse and Alcoholism. *"Alcohol Alert-Relapse and Craving."* www.niaaa.nih.gov, 1989.

National Institute on Alcohol Abuse and Alcoholism. "What You Should Know about Alcohol Problems." *Substance Abuse in Brief* 2:1, 2003.

Norton, V. P. "Interrelationships of nutrition and voluntary alcohol consumption in experimental animals." *British Journal of Addiction* 72:203-12, 1997.

O'Halloren, P. "Pyridine nucleotides in the prevention, diagnosis and treatment of problem drinkers." *Western Journal of Surgery Obstetrics and Gynecology* 69:101-4, 1961.

Oka, H., S. Yamamoto, T. Kuroki, et al. "Perspective study of chemoprevention of hepatocellular carcinoma with sho-saiko-to (TJ-9)." *Cancer* 76:743-9, 1995.

Overstreet, D. H., W. M. Keung, A. H. Rezvani, A. M. Massi, and D. Y. Lee. "Herbal remedies for alcoholism: promises and possible pitfalls." *Alcoholism Clinical and Experimental Research* 27(2):177-85, 2003.

Penninx, B. W, J. M. Guralnik, L. Ferrucci, et al. "Vitamin B (12) deficiency and depression in physically disabled older women: epidemiologic evidence from the Women's Health and Aging Study." *American Journal of Psychiatry* 157:715-21, 2000.

Piras, G., M. Makin, and M. Baba. "Sho-saiko-to, a traditional kampo medicine, enhances the anti-HIV-1 activity of lamivudine (3TC) in vitro." *Microbiology and Immunology* 41:435-9, 1997.

Pittler, M. H., and E. Ernst. "Efficacy of kava extract for treating anxiety: systematic review and meta-analysis." *Journal of Clinical Psychopharmacology* 20:84-89, 2000.

Prabakaran, K., et al. "Control of alcohol addiction by SKV therapy – its action on water, food intake, brain function and cell membrane composition." *Pharmacology Research Communications* 20(2): 99-116, 1988.

Rana, A. C., and Y. Avadhoot. "Hepatoprotective effects of Andrographis paniculata against carbon tetrachloride-induced liver damage." *Archives of Pharmaceutical Research* 14(1):93-5, 1991.

Reid, D. *A Handbook of Chinese Healing Herbs.* Boston: Shambhala Publications, 1995.

Rezvani, A. H., D. H. Overstreet, Y. Yang, and E. Clark Jr. "Attenuation of alcohol intake by extract of Hypericum perforatum (St. John's Wort) in two different strains of alcohol-preferring rats." *Alcohol Alcoholism* 34(5):699-705, 1999.

Rogers, L .L., and R. B. Pelton. "Glutamine in the treatment of alcoholism." *Quarterly Journal of Studies on Alcohol* 18(4):581-587, 1957.

Rogers, L. L., R. B. Pelton, and R. Williams. "Amino acid supplementation and voluntary consumption by rats." *Journal of Biological Chemistry* 220(1):321-323, 1956.

Rogers, L. L., R. B. Pelton, and R. Williams. "Voluntary alcohol consumption by rats following administration of glutamine." *Journal of Biological Chemistry* 214 (2):503-6, 1955.

Rosenfeld, I. "Think Before You Drink." *Parade Magazine* April 6, 2003:8-10.

Ruden, R. *The Craving Brain.* New York: HarperCollins, 1997.

Ryle, P. R., and A. D. Thomson. "Nutrition and vitamins in alcoholism." *Contemporary Issues in Clinical Biochemistry* 1:188-224, 1984.

Sabelli, H. C., J. Fawcett, F. Gustovsky, et al. "Clinical studies on the phenylethylamine hypothesis of affective disorder: urine and blood phenylacetic acid and phenylalanine dietary supplements." *Journal of Clinical Psychiatry* 47:66-70, 1986.

Scheer, J. F. "Evening primrose oil: world-renowned cure-all." *Better Nutrition for Today's Living* 57(2):72, 1995.

Schneider, P. "Which herbs really work?" *New Choices* 38(7):19-30, 1998.

Schuckit, M. A. "Alcohol and Alcoholism," in Fauci, A. S., E. Braunwald, K. J. Isselbacher, et al, eds. *Harrison's Principles of Internal Medicine, 14th ed.* New York: McGraw-Hill, 1998.

Serra, S., G. Vacca, S. Tumatis, A. Carrucciu, P. Morazzoni, E. Bombardelli, G. Colombo, G. L. Gessa, and M. A. Carai. "Anti-relapse properties of IDN 5082, a standardized extract of Salvia miltiorrhiza, in alcohol-preferring rats." *Journal of Ethnopharmacology* 88(2-3):249-52, 2003.

Shanmugasundaram, E. R., and K. R. Shanmugasundaram. "An Indian herbal formula (SKV) for controlling voluntary ethanol intake in rats with chronic alcoholism." *Journal of Ethnopharmacology* 17(2):171-82, 1986.

Shanmugasundaram, E. R., U. Subramaniam, R. Santhini, and K. R. Shanmugasundaram. "Studies on brain structures and neurological function in alcoholic rats controlled by an Indian medicinal formula (SKV)." *Journal of Ethnopharmacology* 17(3):225-45, 1986.

Shu, H. Y. *Oriental Materia Medica: A Concise Guide.* Palos Verdes, CA: Oriental Healing Arts Press, 1986.

Simon, D. *The Wisdom of Healing.* New York: Harmony Books, 1997.

Sinclair, S. "Chinese herbs: A clinical review of astragalus, ligusticum and schizandrae." *Alternative Medicine Review* 3(5):338-344, 1998.

Singh, N., et al. "Withania somnifera – a rejuvenating herbal drug which enhances survival during stress." *International Journal of Crude Drug Research* 1982:20-29.

Singleton, E. G., and D. A. Gorelick. "Mechanisms of alcohol craving and their clinical implications," in Galanter, M., ed. *Recent Developments in Alcoholism: Volume 14. The Consequences of Alcoholism.* New York: Plenum Press, 1998.

Smith, R. F. "A five-year trial of massive nicotinic acid therapy of alcoholics in Michigan." *Journal of Orthomolecular Psychiatry* 3:327-31, 1974.

Smith, R. F. "Status report concerning the use of megadose nicotinic acid in alcoholics." *Journal of Orthomolecular Psychiatry* 7(1), 1978.

Sonnebichler, J., and I. Zetl. "Stimulating influence of flavonolignan derivative on proliferation, RNA synthesis and protein synthesis in liver cells," in Okolicsanyi, L., G. Csomos, and G. Crespaldi, eds. *Assessment and Management of Hepatobiliary Disease.* Berlin: Springer-Verlag, 1987.

Spivey, A. "Sobering effects from the lowly kudzu." *Endeavors Magazine* University of North Carolina at Chapel Hill, April, 1996.

Steiner, G. G. "Kava as an anticraving agent: preliminary data." *Pacific Health Dialog* 8(2):335-9, 2001.

Sukul, N. C., S. Ghost, S. P. Sinhababu, and A. Sukul. "Strychnos nux-vomica extract and its ultra-high dilution reduce voluntary ethanol intake in rats." *Journal of Alternative and Complementary Medicine* 7(2):187-93, 2001.

Sukul, A., P. Sarkar, S. P. Sinhababu, and N. C. Sukul. "Altered solution structure of alcoholic medium of potentized Nux vomica underlies its antialcoholic effect." *Homeopathy* 89(2):73-77, 2000.

Svoboda, R. *Ayurveda Life, Health and Longevity.* New York: Penguin USA, 1993

Teeguarden, R. *Radiant Health.* New York: Warner Books, 1998.

Television News Service/Medical Breakthroughs Ivanoe Broadcast News, Inc. "A Natural Cure for Alcoholism." #1246, 1998.

Tiffany, S. T. "Cognitive Concepts of Craving." *Alcohol Research & Health* 23(3), 1999.

Tiffany, S. T., and C. A, Conklin. "A cognitive processing model of alcohol craving and compulsive alcohol use." *Addiction* 95(2):S145-S153, 2000.

Trunnell, J. B., and J. I. Wheeler. "Preliminary report on experiments with orally administered glutamine in treatment of alcoholism." *Journal of the American Chemistry Society* Houston, December, 1955.

Tuchweber, B., R. Sieck, and W. Trost. "Prevention by silibinin of phalloidin induced hepatotoxicity." *Toxicology and Applied Pharmacology* 51:265-75, 1979.

University of North Carolina at Chapel Hill. "Study Finds St. John's Wort Can Cut Alcohol Consumption." Press Release, June 6, 1998.

U. S. Departments of Agriculture and Health and Human Services. *Dietary Guidelines for Americans-Fifth Edition.* Home and Garden Bulletin 232, 2000.

U. S. Food and Drug Administration Center for Food Safety and Applied Nutrition. *Economic Characterization of the Dietary Supplement Industry Final Report.* www.cfsan.fda.gov, March, 1999.

Utrilla, M .P., A. Zarzuelo, S. Risco, et al. "Isolation of the saikosaponin responsible for the anti-inflammatory activity of Bupleurum gibralticum Lam root extract." *Phytotherapy Research* 5:43-5, 1991.

Walsh, N. "Milk thistle for liver disease." *Family Practice News* 32(1):8, 2002.

Weil, A. *Natural Health, Natural Medicine.* Boston: Houghton Mifflin Co, 1990.

Werbach, M. R. "Alcohol craving." *International Journal of Alternative and Complementary Medicine* July:32, 1993.

Werbach, M. R. *Healing through Nutrition.* New York: HarperCollins, 1993.

Werbach, M. R. *Nutritional Influences on Illness, 3rd ed.* Tarzana, CA: Third Line Press, 1999.

Williams, R. J. *Alcoholism: The Nutritional Approach.* Austin: University of Texas Press, 1958.

Williams, R. J. *Nutrition Against Disease.* New York: Pitman Press, 1971.

Zal, M. "Five herbs for depression, anxiety, and sleep disorders: uses, benefits and adverse effects." *Consultant* 39(12):3343, 1999.

Printed in the United States
125312LV00002B/65/A